QUICK & EASY pilates

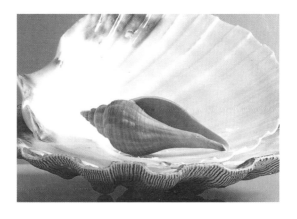

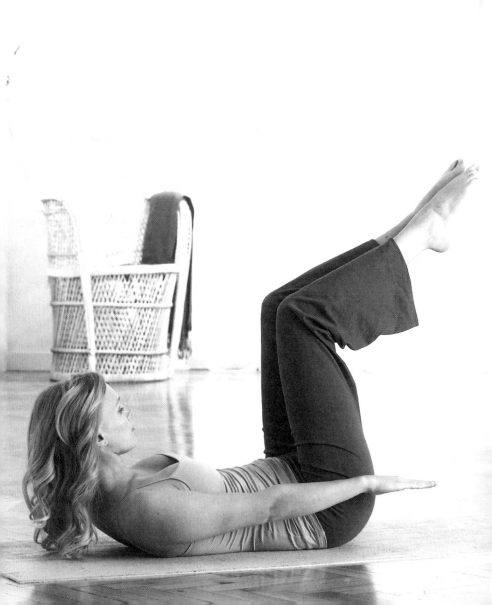

DUNCAN BAIRD PUBLISHERS

LONDON

QUICK & EASY pilates

Karen Smith

5-minute routines for

anyone

anytime

anywhere

QUICK
&EASY pilates
Karen Smith

First published in the United Kingdom and Ireland in 2008 by
Duncan Baird Publishers Ltd
Sixth Floor
Castle House
75–76 Wells Street
London WIT 3QH

Conceived, created and designed by Duncan Baird Publishers

Copyright © Duncan Baird Publishers 2008
Text copyright © Karen Smith 2008
Photography copyright © Duncan Baird Publishers 2008

Managing Editor: Grace Cheetham
Editor: Zoë Fargher
Managing Designer: Manisha Patel
Designer: Jantje Doughty
Commissioned photography: Jules Selmes

British Library Cataloguing-in-Publication Data:
A CIP record for this book is available from the British Library

ISBN: 978-1-84483-657-4

10 9 8 7 6 5 4 3 2 1

Typeset in Gill Sans, Nofret and Helvetica Neue
Colour reproduction by Scanhouse, Malaysia
Printed in China by Imago

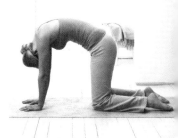

I would like to dedicate this book to
all those I have taught. It is you who
have taught me.

contents

6 introduction

anytime

22 morning wake-up
24 lunchtime stretch
26 afternoon uplifter
28 evening de-stress
30 bedtime wind-down
32 lazy weekend
34 before a night out
36 before a meeting
38 at a conference

anywhere

42 in your bedroom
44 on your sofa
46 in your dining room
48 in your bathroom
50 in the park
54 on the beach
56 at your desk
58 on a plane
60 in your car
62 in a hotel room

stress busters

66 body relaxer
68 neck reliever
70 shoulder loosener
72 arm releaser
74 back soother
76 lower-body easer
78 all-over calmer

energy boosters

82 all-over energizer
84 tummy lifter
86 spine reviver
88 tummy refresher
90 body booster
92 thigh invigorator
94 outer-thigh lifter

toners and strengtheners

98 body toner
100 posture enhancer
102 waist tightener
104 tummy booster
106 pelvic-floor firmer
108 tummy flattener
110 butt enhancer
112 hip toner
114 thigh firmer
116 hamstring helper
118 spine strengthener
120 back rebuilder
122 upper-arm restorer

124 everyday sequences
126 index
128 acknowledgments

introduction

Pilates is a carefully structured system of exercises that co-ordinates the movement of muscles with the breathing. It tones all the body's muscle groups and improves posture, muscle definition and strength.

The founder of the Pilates system, Joseph Pilates, was born in Dusseldorf, Germany in 1880. A fragile and unhealthy child, as he grew to adulthood, Pilates took a systematic approach to improving his physical fitness. He experimented with martial arts, yoga and meditation, as well as traditional aerobic sports and strength conditioning. He realized that by integrating these techniques, and using his mind and body in unison, he could strengthen his deep postural muscles to condition his entire body and improve his overall well-being. His system was so effective that, despite his early years of poor health, Pilates became a keen sportsman, a gymnast, a skier, a boxer and a circus performer.

Pilates moved to England in 1912, where he was interned at the beginning of World War 1. Helping out in the camp infirmary, he experimented with attaching springs to hospital beds so that, as they recuperated, patients could tone and stretch their muscles through resistance exercises. His techniques were hugely successful. After the war, Pilates returned to Germany and then in 1926 emigrated to the USA. With his wife Clara, he set up a studio in New York that quickly began to attract dancers, actors, athletes and gymnasts. Pilates called his revolutionary new bodywork method "contrology". His regime, which after his death in 1967 became known simply as Pilates, has now been practised for more than eighty years. However, it is only during the last twenty years that Pilates has become a mainstream form of exercise, with classes timetabled at fitness clubs, and independent teachers offering sessions on a private or group basis. Medical professionals, osteopaths and physiotherapists have also realized the efficacy of the Pilates system and now use it to prevent or rehabilitate injuries, enabling Pilates to provide a complementary addition to their treatment.

who is Pilates for?

Anyone who wishes to improve their total fitness, posture and appearance will benefit from practising Pilates exercises. Pilates focuses on the body as a whole, and on working with people as individuals. Its versatility means that practitioners can adapt the exercises to their own needs on a day-to-day or week-to-week basis. With Pilates, it is less about "what" you do, and more about "how" you do it.

Whether you are a first-time exerciser, are elderly, or simply need to break out of a sedentary lifestyle, Pilates offers a safe, effective form of exercise for all ages and fitness levels. The system is also widely used by professional sports people, athletes, dancers, musicians and other performers for whom good posture is vital. It can be of particular benefit to anyone suffering from RSI (repetitive strain injury), and those wishing to prevent or alleviate osteoporosis. Pilates is also especially useful for those suffering from chronic back pain, or pain in the neck and shoulders (see pages 10–11).

core stability

The aim of the Pilates system is to create strength and stability in your body's core in order to protect your lower back while your limbs move freely. The core of your body is the part between your pelvis and your ribcage – your abdomen. Four large muscles wrap around your abdomen, which hold your internal organs in place. The stronger these muscles are, the more support they will provide for your body.

Imagine that a corset has been laced up tightly around your middle. This is the support that you should always feel around your abdomen and back when you are practising Pilates. Engaging your pelvic floor muscles (the muscles that you "hold" to stop yourself urinating) at the same time will stabilize your pelvis, making your whole body firmer and stronger. Once you get the feel for using these core muscles, you will be able to use their strength to help you stand, sit and move properly, giving you better overall posture.

8

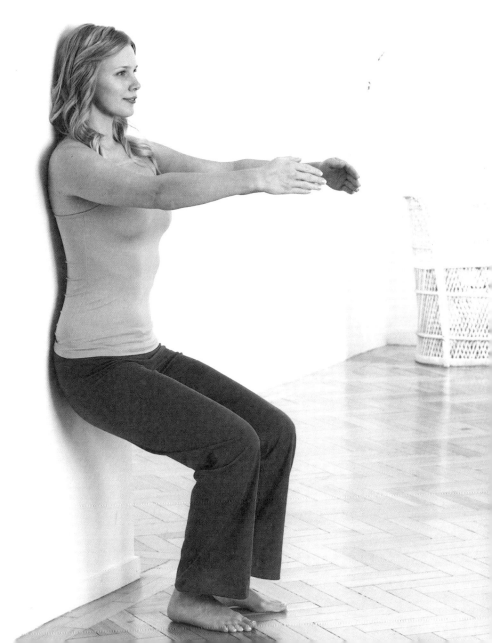

what are the benefits of Pilates?

Practised regularly, Pilates can restore joint flexibility, increase the efficiency of your circulatory system and tone slack muscles. As you strengthen your body, you may find that your levels of stress decrease. And as your body awareness grows, you'll notice that your posture, co-ordination, balance and alignment all improve, giving you a feeling of confidence and of being "grounded" in your body. As this correct posture and alignment will also allow your body to function more efficiently, you'll probably find that posture-related headaches and other aches and pains will disappear. Finally, on a purely physical level, strengthening the core abdominals will give you a flatter stomach!

Pilates for back, shoulder and neck pain

Around eighty per cent of my Pilates clients came to me because they suffered from back, neck or shoulder pain. I myself began Pilates because I sustained a serious neck injury in a car accident. Perhaps you too have picked up or bought this book because you are suffering from back, neck or shoulder pain, or know someone who is.

Back pain ranks alongside the common cold as a primary reason why we take sick days off work. And although some back pain occurs as a result of injury, whether from sports or an accident, the way we use our bodies on a daily basis causes far more. For example, if you sit at a desk for hours each day, your upper body can become tired, and develop stiffness in the joints and tension in the muscles. In the long term this can be detrimental to the skeletal and muscular condition of your whole body, commonly leading to back pain.

Furthermore, it may surprise you to know that many back problems are caused by weakness in the abdominal muscles. Weak abdominals can't properly support your back, which puts your spinal column and back muscles under strain. To strengthen your abdominals, and thus improve your posture and relieve the pressure on your back, you need to replace repetitive, harmful patterns of posture and movement with others that are safer for your body. This takes time and effort, as it involves developing greater conscious – and subconscious – awareness of your body and how it functions.

The Pilates system is designed to improve all aspects of your body awareness by helping you to achieve precision in the control of your muscles, in your co-ordination and in your fluidity of movement. In these ways Pilates is wonderful at helping to overcome chronic back pain, and any associated muscular or joint pain, such as that in your neck and shoulders. Many of my clients who started Pilates because of back pain are helped purely by working on the principle of core stability.

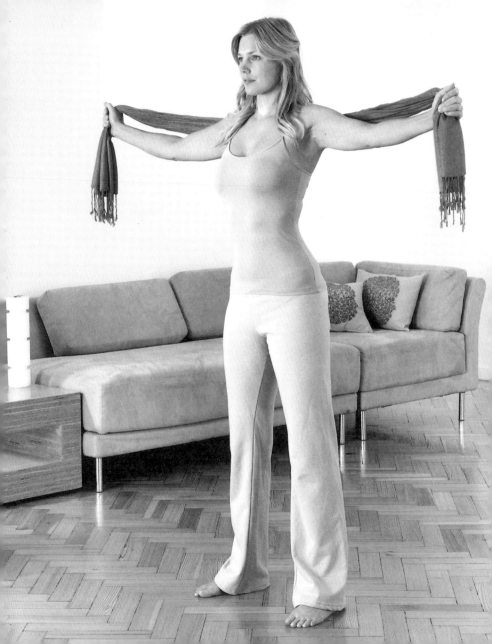

the eight principles of Pilates

Joseph Pilates based his system on eight essential principles:

- **Relaxation** Through relaxation you will become aware of where you hold tension – this varies from person to person and depends on your lifestyle. Once you are aware of where you store tension, you can use your Pilates practice to release tense muscles and improve mobility and flexibility. The secret lies in knowing how to work the relevant area, without tensing the surrounding muscles.

- **Concentration** Pilates exercises aim to train both mind and body: Pilates himself said "It is the mind itself which builds the body." Ideally, each Pilates movement should originate in your mind. This way you can really "feel" a movement as you practise it, rather than just executing the exercise mechanically. With your mind and body focused together, and working in synergy, you can develop an awareness of what you are doing with every part of your body.

- **Alignment** The next principle is that you must bring your body into correct alignment. This is essential if you want to get the right muscles working to support a joint, not stress it. Whether you are standing, sitting, or lying down, always visualize your body like a series of building blocks – your head should sit directly over your ribcage, which sits over your pelvis, which sits over each leg, which each sit over a foot.

13

- **Breathing** Lateral, or thoracic, breathing is the key to Pilates. It will maximize the use of the lower part of the lungs, increasing your oxygen intake. The timing of the breath is integral to the timing of the exercises, as you can help or hinder a movement by breathing in or out. See pages 15–16 for more details on how to breathe correctly.

- **Centering** Your body's centre of gravity is in the abdominal cavity, just below your navel. According to Pilates' theory, all movement should originate from this strong, stable core. With your central muscles engaged, you free your body to move in a more harmonious way.

- **Co-ordination** This principle works alongside concentration. Your mind should work slightly ahead of your body so that you always know in advance what the next movement will be and how to co-ordinate your breathing with it. With practice you will be able to practise whole series of co-ordinated and balanced movements.

- **Flowing movements** Pilates movements are generally slow and controlled, lengthening away from a strong centre. Slow doesn't mean easy, though – quite the opposite. You need precision and strength, and it is less easy to cheat! The aim is to move through each exercise efficiently, maintaining the flow and rhythm of movement.

- **Stamina** With regular Pilates practice, the endurance of your postural muscles will improve. As you become stronger, you will no longer

14

waste energy holding tension in your muscles, but will be able to harness that energy as physical stamina for sports, everyday actions and general fitness. Your mental stamina will improve, too.

breathing correctly

Joseph Pilates cautioned that when practising his exercises "Above all, learn how to breathe correctly." He devised a particular way to breathe that is known as lateral, or thoracic, breathing. In this form of breathing, as you inhale you expand your entire ribcage (back, sides and front) without relaxing your abdomen. By expanding the whole ribcage, you increase the volume of your lungs and your intake of oxygen. This also strengthens the muscles between your ribs.

During Pilates exercises, you should always breathe in through your nose and out through your mouth. As a general rule, breathe in to prepare for a movement, then breathe out while you engage your muscles and move. Then, breathe in again to recover. By moving on the exhalation, you will be able to relax into the stretch. You will also stabilize your core during the hardest part of the exercise.

Don't worry if you find it difficult to breathe in this way. Correct breathing will take time to master, but will eventually become second nature. Here are a few simple guidelines to help you practise:

15

- **Inhalation** Place both hands just under your breastbone with your middle fingers touching. As you breathe in, keep your shoulders and chest muscles relaxed. Breathe deeply into your mid-back (your finger tips should part slightly). This is a proper in-breath. During Pilates practice imagine your lungs like bellows inflating as you inhale. Your ribcage should expand laterally (sideways). If you are wearing a bra, imagine the strap widening. Don't force your inhalation though.
- **Exhalation** As you breathe out, ensure that your shoulders and chest muscles remain relaxed (the middle fingers of your hands should come back to touching each other). During Pilates practice, if you are lying down, allow your body to sink into the floor. Visualize your lungs like bellows deflating. Feel your ribs closing back together and your chest softening. Release any tension between your shoulder blades. Allow your out-breath to be full and relaxed.

contraindications

Consult your medical practitioner before you start Pilates exercises, especially if you are pregnant or undergoing medical treatment. Avoid exercising if you have just eaten a meal or drunk alcohol, if you are feeling unwell, or if you have taken painkillers. If you are recovering from an injury, consult your physical therapist before practising Pilates.

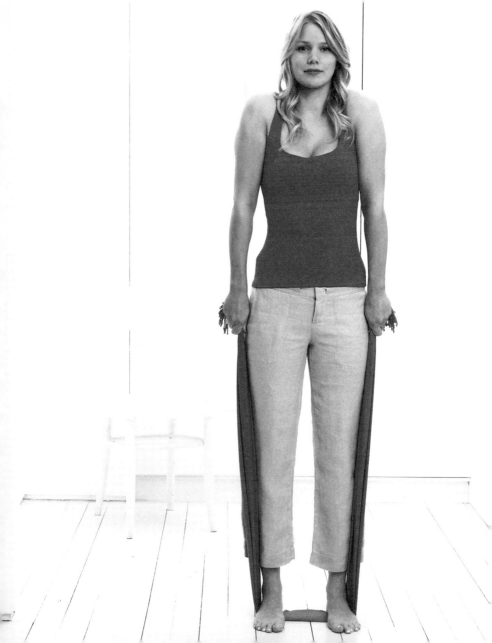

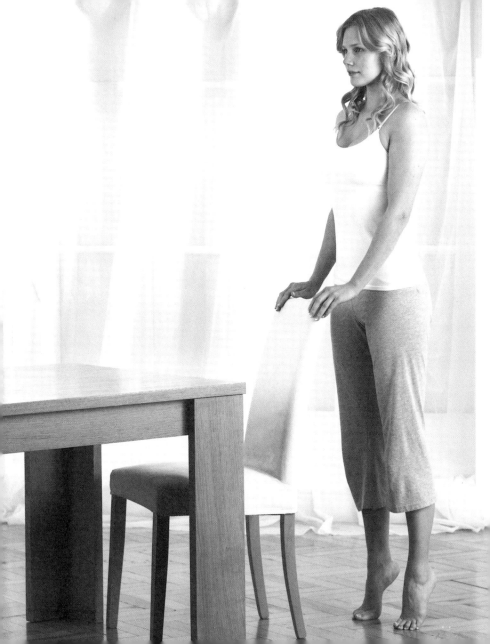

how to use this book

Before you start exercising, read the sections on breathing (pages 15–16) and core stability (page 8), as they will provide a good foundation for you to build upon. For Chapter 1, I have chosen various exercises that I think are particularly good for certain times of the day (although don't let this stop you practising them at other times of day, too!). You don't need lots of space to practise Pilates, and Chapter 2 suggests locations that make practising really accessible – such as in your car or while your kids are playing in the park. Chapter 3 contains exercises to de-stress the body, while Chapter 4 offers more energetic exercises that will pep you up if you are feeling lethargic. Finally, the last chapter will help you to tone and strengthen specific areas of your body.

As you become stronger, you can try different combinations of exercises. If you need guidance, refer to the Everyday Sequences section on pages 124–125 to help you get started.

I healed my own body by practising Pilates and this inspired me to become a teacher. I love the fact that the versatility of Pilates allows me to tailor a program to every client's specific needs. Proceed at your own pace, and soon you will discover how quickly and easily Pilates can create balance in your life and improve your well-being.

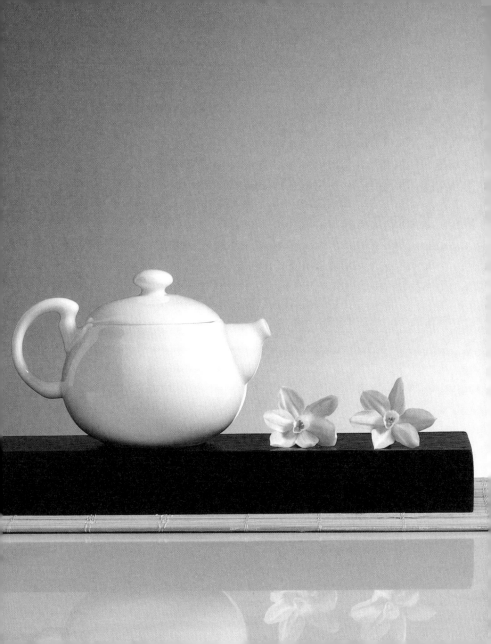

anytime

Have you ever woken up feeling stiff? Pilates first thing in the morning can liberate your body for the day ahead. If you have a sedentary job, a Pilates exercise at lunchtime can alleviate back strain. In the evening, a soothing twist will help you to unwind and release accumulated tension. In short, you can practise Pilates any time.

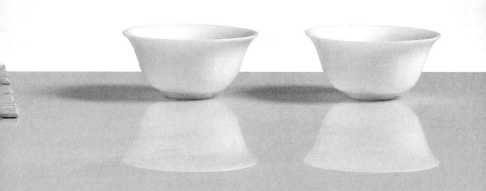

morning wake-up
activating

loosen your back before you start your day

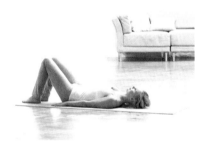 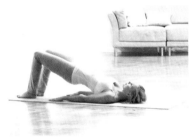

1 Lie on your back with both knees bent, feet placed hip-width apart. Rest your arms by your sides with your palms facing down. Ground your feet by visualizing three points of connection to the floor: your heels, your big toes and your little toes. Relax the back of your shoulders.

2 Breathe in, and as you breathe out pull in your abdominals and start to tilt your pelvis so that your pubic bone lifts upward. Keeping your buttocks strong, continue to curl your lower spine away from the floor. Maintain a smooth movement and lift your spine higher until your mid-back is elevated, too.

22

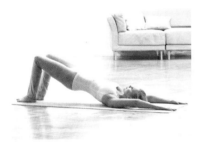

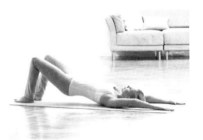

3 Breathe in and raise your arms. Pull your shoulders down into your back and lift your arms, moving them backward until they rest on the floor behind your head. Feel a long stretch that reaches from your fingertips all the way to your knees.

4 As you breathe out, slowly curl your spine down, vertebra by vertebra, keeping your abdominals pulled in to help you control your spine. Once your tailbone is on the floor, bring your arms back down by your sides. Repeat this exercise seven times.

23

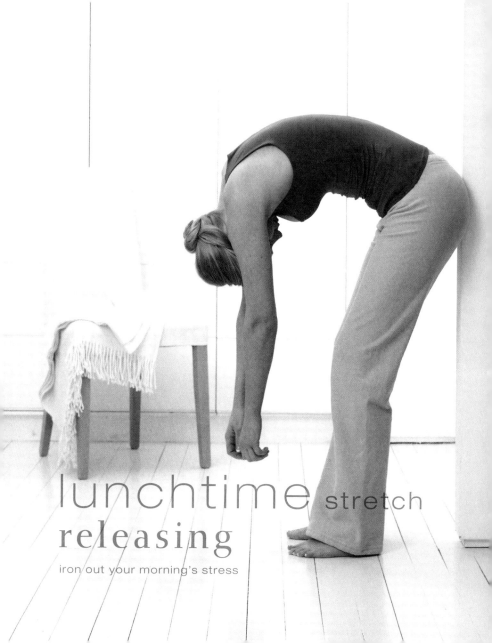

lunchtime stretch
releasing
iron out your morning's stress

1 Stand with your back against a wall and place your feet slightly in front of the line of your hips, about the length of one of your own feet away from the wall. The backs of your shoulders and your hips rest against the wall, and your head is in line with your neck and spine.

2 Breathe in without lifting your shoulders. As you breathe out, nod your head forward, pulling in your abdominals. Start to roll your spine forward, keeping your tailbone connected to the wall. Imagine your spine is a wheel turning and each vertebra is a spoke of the wheel.

3 (*left*) Continue rolling down until your hands are about 10–15cm (4–6in) away from the floor. Your arms should hang loosely from your shoulders and your head should feel heavy. Gently shake your head from side to side and swing your arms a little to make sure there is no tension in your neck or shoulders.

4 Breathe in, then as you breathe out start to roll your spine back up. Use your abdominals to press each vertebra against the wall. Drop your tailbone toward the floor. Continue rolling your spine up, pulling your shoulders down into your back. Repeat this exercise seven times.

1 Stand with your feet hip-width apart. Your shoulders should be directly over your hips. Relax your arms down by your sides and hold a stretch band or scarf between your hands, which should be slightly wider than shoulder-width apart. Pull in your abdominals and bend your knees slightly to prevent the joints from locking.

2 (*right*) Breathe in as you lift your arms to shoulder height, being careful not to raise your shoulders. Continue to lift your arms above your head. If you are using a stretch band, it should remain slack at this stage even though your arms are outstretched.

3 Breathe out and stretch the band, or move your hands toward the ends of the scarf, so that your arms are much further apart. Bend your elbows a little and pull the band or scarf down behind your back, until you feel a stretch across the front of your chest and shoulders.

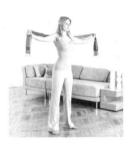

4 Breathe in and raise your arms over your head. Keep your abdominals engaged to prevent your back from arching, and be careful not to poke your head forward. Breathe out and bring your arms back down to the starting position in front of you, allowing your arms to hang loosely from your shoulders. Repeat the whole exercise seven times.

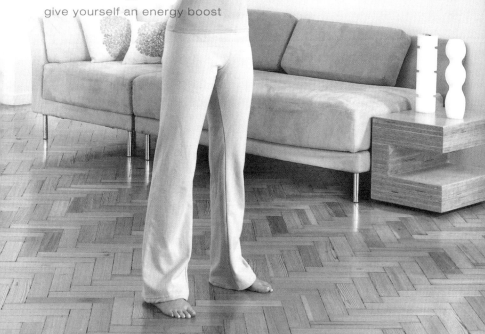

afternoon uplifter
invigorating
give yourself an energy boost

evening de-stress
unwinding

release your legs with a well-earned stretch

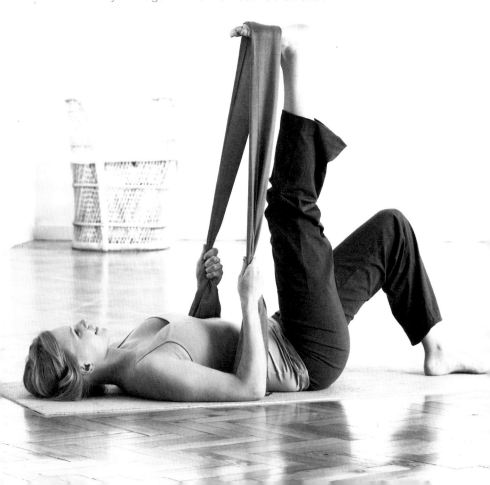

1

Lie on your back with both knees bent and your feet flat on the floor, hip-width apart. Bend your right knee toward your chest and place a stretch band or scarf over the sole of your foot. Rest your upper arms on the floor so that your shoulders are relaxed. Pull in your abdominals and release your spine toward the floor.

2

Breathe in, then as you breathe out extend your right leg forward at a 45-degree angle to the floor, pushing your foot away from you. Be careful not to lock your knee. Flex your ankle so that your toes are pointing over your head.

3

(*left*) Still breathing out, continue to raise your leg, pulling the band or scarf toward your chest until you feel a slight stretch at the back of your thigh. You may also feel a stretch behind your knee. Ensure that you keep your tailbone on the floor, so that your pelvis does not lift.

4

Breathe in as you bend your knee halfway toward your chest. Feel your hamstring muscles release and relax, then extend your leg forward and pull it upward to repeat the stretch. Keep your shoulder blades relaxed during the whole exercise. Practise this exercise eight times with your right leg, and eight with your left.

1   Lie on your left side with your head on a cushion. Ensure that your head and spine are in a straight line. Bend your knees to a 45-degree angle with your hips, and position your right hip directly over your left. Stretch your arms out at shoulder height, with your palms together.

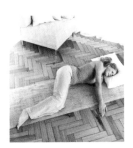

2   Breathe in and lift your right arm up toward the ceiling, turning your head gently to look at it. Bend your right elbow slightly to prevent the joint from locking. Draw your right shoulder down away from your ear. Pull in your abdominals to help your pelvis remain stable.

3   (*right*) Breathe out and rotate your upper spine, enabling your right arm to open further out. Continue to turn your head, following your hand with your eyes. Be careful not to strain your neck. Breathe in and start to bring your right arm back over your body.

4   Breathe out and bring your right hand to rest back on top of your left. Let the left side of your head completely relax into the cushion. Repeat this exercise three further times with your right arm, then turn over to practise it four times in all with your left.

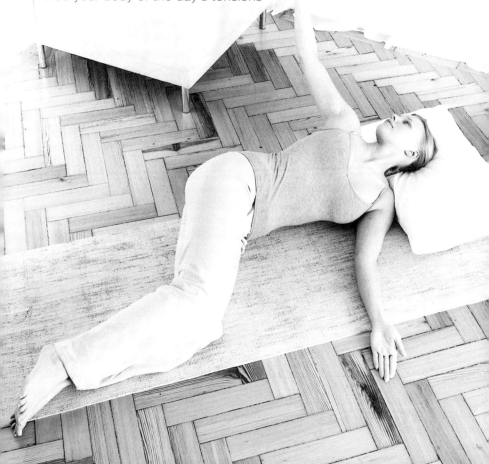

bedtime wind-down

soothing

free your body of the day's tensions

lazy weekend strengthening

enrich your time off with these flowing movements

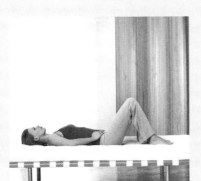

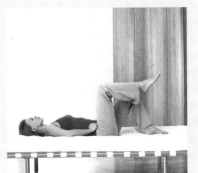

1 Lie on your back with both knees bent, feet placed hip-width apart. Place your hands on your hips to stabilize them. Relax your back so that there is a small natural curve and a gap under your lower spine.

2 Breathe in and bend your right knee toward your chest so that it is directly over your hip. Softly point your right toes away from you, and pull in your abdominals to help keep your pelvis still and stable.

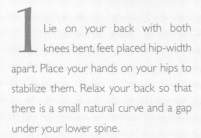

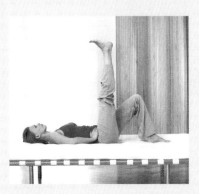 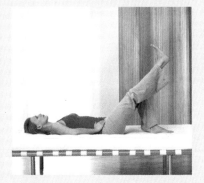

3 Breathe out as you straighten and extend your leg upward, keeping your tailbone down and the back of your hips heavy. Breathe in and flex your ankle so that your heel is moving upward and your toes are pointing behind you. You should feel a stretch in the back of your calf.

4 Breathe out and, keeping your leg stretched, lower it slowly and with control. Take your leg to about 15cm (6in) off the floor, using the strength of your abdominals to prevent your lower back from arching. From this position, bend your knee toward your chest to repeat steps 2–4. Practise this exercise eight times on each side.

33

before a night out
energizing

feel strong and revitalized

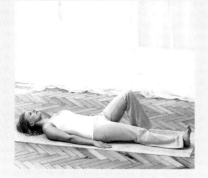
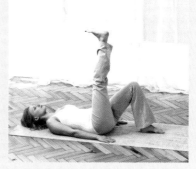

1 Lie on your back with your left knee bent and your right leg extended on the ground. Relax your arms by your sides with your palms facing down. Flex your right ankle so that your toes are pointing upward. Engage your abdominals.

2 Breathe in and lift your right leg straight up, keeping your hips still and your buttocks connected to the floor. Make sure your shoulders stay relaxed and the backs of your hips remain grounded. Lift your leg as high as you can with your knee straight.

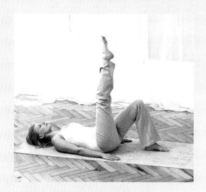 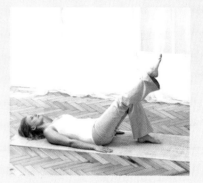

3 Keeping your knee straight, point the toes of your right foot. Look up at your foot to check that it is pointing in a straight line from your knee, and not twisting inward from your ankle.

4 Breathe out and begin to lower your leg with the control and support of your abdominals. Making sure that your back doesn't arch, continue to lower your leg to about 15cm (6in) off the floor. Flex your right ankle again, ready to repeat steps 2–4. Practise this exercise eight times on each side.

35

1 Stand with your legs hip-width apart. Place a stretch band or long scarf under your feet, and hold on to the ends. Check that your head is aligned over your spine. Draw your shoulders down into your back. Relax your neck and pull in your abdominals.

2 (*right*) Breathe in. As you breathe out, slowly and gently turn your head to the right so that your face is in profile. Your shoulders and hips remain still. Breathe in and bring your head back to the centre, then breathe out and turn your head to the left. Breathe in again and bring your head back to the centre. Breathe out.

3 As you breathe in again, raise your shoulders up toward your ears. Breathe out and slide your shoulder blades back down toward the back of your ribcage. Feel as if your neck has grown longer and that you are releasing all the tension from your neck and shoulder area.

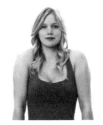

4 Repeat steps 2 and 3 three times, turning your head to alternate sides. Then, on the fourth time, replace the shoulder lift in step three with shoulder circles. As you breathe in, circle your shoulders up and forward, and as you exhale, slide your shoulder blades down into your back. Practise this three times circling forward, and three times backward.

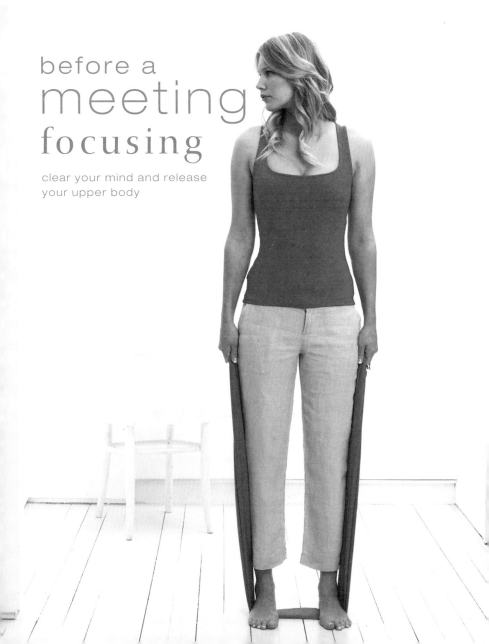

before a
meeting
focusing

clear your mind and release
your upper body

at a
conference
balancing

re-centre yourself with a gentle twist

1 Sit on a chair with your buttocks close to the edge of the seat, feet placed firmly hip-width apart on the floor. Fold your arms in front of you, in line with your upper chest. Release your shoulders down. Keep your neck relaxed and pull in your abdominals. Breathe in and lengthen up through your spine.

2 (*opposite*) Breathe out and start to turn your body to your right. Make sure that you initiate the movement from your spine, and not from your shoulders or your arms. Your hips remain still and facing forward, your arms stay at chest height.

3 Breathe in and bring your upper body back to the starting position. Pull in your abdominals again, and lift your pelvic floor muscles. This will enable you to sit higher on your "sit" bones, which will help you to achieve a stronger, deeper twist in your spine.

4 Breathe out to turn your body to your left. This time, imagine the top of your head reaching an extra 2.5cm (1in) up toward the ceiling. Support the back of your body by imagining a zip fastening from your pubic bone up toward your navel and onward to your breastbone. Repeat this exercise five times.

39

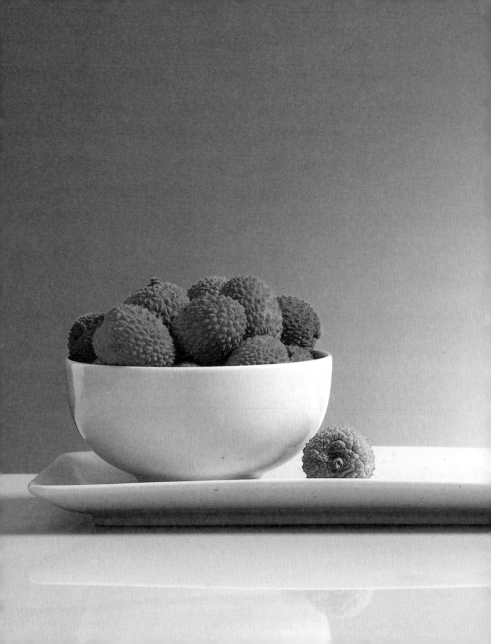

anywhere

You don't always need to attend a Pilates class to get the benefits of

Pilates practice. You can practise the simple exercises in this chapter

wherever you are – indoors or outdoors, at home or at work. Whether

you prefer to stand up, or sit or lie down, these exercises will energize,

strengthen and relax your whole body.

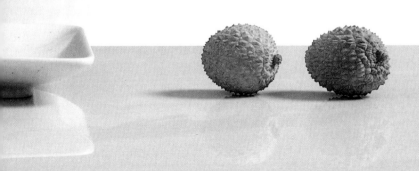

in your bedroom
relaxing

open and release your lower back

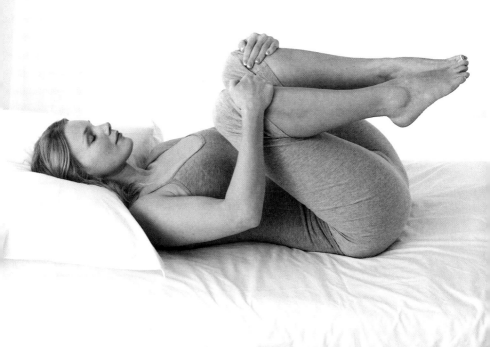

1 Lie on your bed with your legs stretched out and your arms by your sides. Close your eyes. Inhale, and as you exhale, relax your head into your pillow. Focus on relaxing the back of your neck, shoulders, spine and hips in turn. Gradually release all the tension from your body.

2 (*opposite*) Now turn your attention to your abdomen and gently pull in your stomach, without losing the relaxation in your spine. Breathe in, then as you exhale bring your left and then your right knee to your chest. Breathing normally, hold your legs just below each knee joint and allow your knees to open.

3 Breathe in again, then as you breathe out pull your knees closer to your chest. Keep your abdominals engaged and your shoulders as relaxed as possible. Feel your lower back and hips release. Continue to breathe normally and hold this position for about one minute.

4 Bring your knees together, then as you breathe out pull them toward your chest one more time. Carefully lower your right and then your left leg, engaging your abdominals to prevent your spine and pelvis from losing their stability.

43

on your sofa
refreshing

awaken your whole body by stimulating your feet

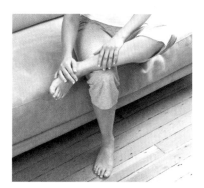

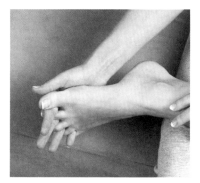

1 Sitting comfortably on a chair, cross your left foot over your right knee. Open and relax your left knee as much as possible. Support your left shin with your left hand, and rest your right hand lightly on your left foot, relaxing your fingers on your ankle.

2 Place the index finger of your right hand between your left big toe and the next toe. Continue to place each of your fingers between your toes, aiming to get the bases of your fingers down to the bases of your toes. If this feels a little awkward, use some hand cream or body lotion to help your fingers slide between your toes.

44

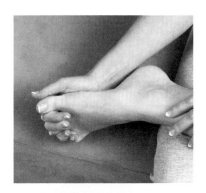

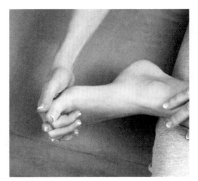

3 Wrap your fingers over the top of your foot and support the arch with the heel of your hand. Now use your fingers to pull your foot forward so that your toes are pointed and your foot arches. You should feel a stretch on the top of your instep.

4 Now, using the heel of your hand to support the ball of your foot, move your toes so that they are bending backward a little. Release your fingers and stand on your left foot; notice how different it feels compared with your right foot. Practise this exercise ten times with each foot.

45

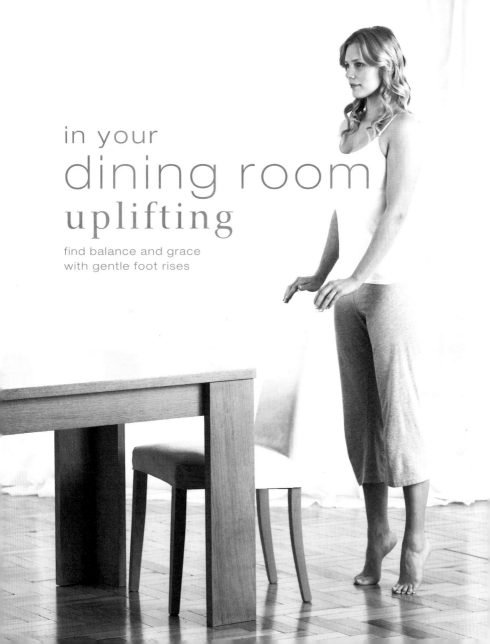

in your
dining room
uplifting

find balance and grace
with gentle foot rises

1 Stand behind a chair in your dining room or kitchen. Place your feet about 30cm (1ft) apart and parallel. Lightly hold on to the back of the chair to steady your balance. Breathe in and lengthen up through your spine. Imagine someone pulling you up from the top of your head.

2 (*opposite*) As you breathe out, shift your weight forward onto the balls of your feet and rise up onto your toes. As you move into this position, you will feel your calf muscles tightening and a stretch in the fronts of your feet and ankles.

3 Breathe in and sense your centre of balance. Check that your weight is distributed equally between your feet. Keep your abdominals engaged to maintain your strong centre. Carefully release one hand to test your balance, and then replace it on the back of the chair.

4 Breathe out as you slowly lower your heels back down, still maintaining the length in your spine. Repeat the whole exercise ten times. To finish, bend your knees slightly to release your calf muscles and stretch your Achilles' tendons.

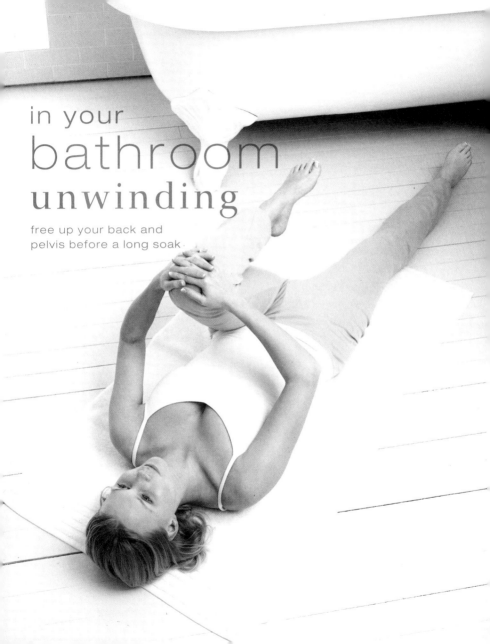

in your
bathroom
unwinding

free up your back and
pelvis before a long soak

1 Lie on the floor on your back, with your legs stretched out and relaxed. Pull in your abdominals to prevent your lower back from arching. Relax your shoulders and draw your shoulder blades down into your back.

2 As you breathe in, carefully pick up your left leg, bending the knee up to your chest. Clasp your hands just below the knee, or at the back of your thigh if you have a knee problem. Imagine dropping your left thigh bone down into your hip joint.

3 (*left*) Breathe out, and stretch and lengthen your right leg along the floor. Breathe in again, and pull the raised knee as far as you can toward your chest to flex your hip. Keep your abdominals strong to help stabilize your pelvis. Hold this position for a count of ten, breathing normally.

4 Breathe out and release your left leg down to the floor, then breathe in and pick up your right leg to repeat the stretch. Pull your thigh toward your chest without tensing your shoulders. Practise this exercise five times with each leg.

in the park
exhilarating

reach up to the sun and refresh your body

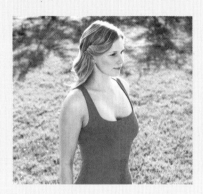 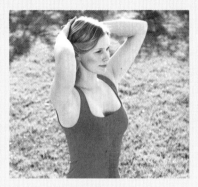

1 Stand with your back straight, feet placed hip-width apart. Relax your shoulder blades down into your back. Your arms are hanging comfortably by your sides, palms facing inward. Visualize your head balancing lightly at the top of your spine.

2 To prepare, breathe in and lengthen up through your spine. Allow your tailbone to drop downward. Breathe out, draw in your abdominals and allow your arms to float upward, extended out to the sides. Clasp your hands at the back of your head.

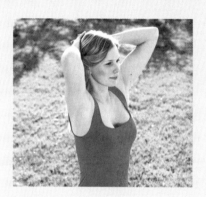 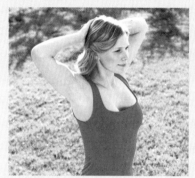

3 Breathe in as you lift your shoulders up to your ears. Breathe out and drop your shoulders down; imagine that they are really heavy. Repeat this shrug, breathing in as you lift your shoulders, then breathing out as you drop them heavily down.

4 Breathe in and gently bring your elbows a little behind your head, keeping them within your peripheral vision. Your shoulder blades will pull toward each other. Release, and repeat this movement three times, breathing in between repetitions. Be careful not to allow your back to arch.

51

in the park

(continued)

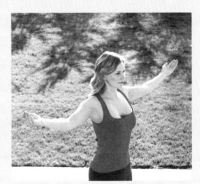 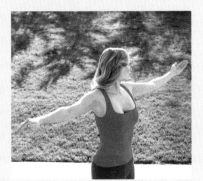

5 Breathe out and unclasp your hands. With your palms facing up, engage the muscles beneath your shoulder blades to slowly open your arms in a wide semi-circle, bringing them down to just below shoulder height. Ensure your elbows remain soft.

6 Breathe in, then as you breathe out isolate your right arm from your shoulder and rotate your arm inward, so that your palm faces down. Simultaneously, turn your head to the left. Keep your right shoulder down.

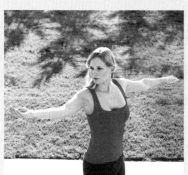

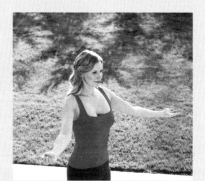

7 Breathe in and rotate your right arm back to the original position with your palm facing up, as you turn your head so that you are looking forward. Breathe out, isolate your left arm from your shoulder and rotate it inward as you turn your head to the right.

8 Breathe in and rotate your left arm back to the original position, simultaneously turning your head to look forward again. As you breathe out, bring both arms down to your sides. Practise the whole exercise five times.

53

on the beach
nurturing
feel grounded and calm

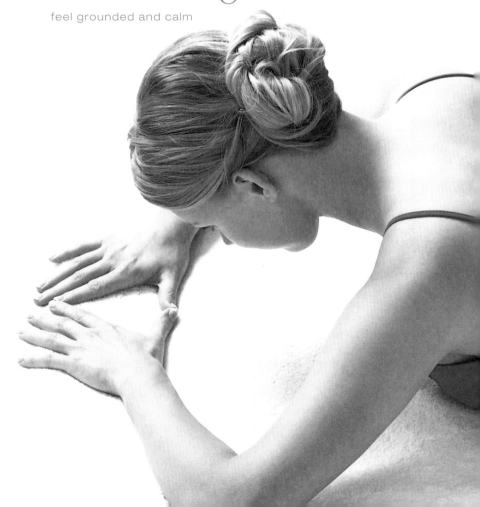

1 Lie on a mat or beach towel on your front, feet hip-width apart and parallel. If you have lower-back problems, place a folded towel under your stomach. Place the tips of your index fingers and thumbs together just above your forehead, making a diamond shape with your arms. Keep your shoulder blades relaxed.

2 (*opposite*) Breathe in, then as you breathe out slide your shoulder blades down into the back of your ribs. Pull in your abdominals to protect your lower back, and lift your upper body about 10cm (4in) away from the floor. Keep your eyes on the floor so that your neck remains long.

3 Stay in this position as you breathe in, feeling the muscles between your shoulder blades working. Imagine the crown of your head lengthening forward and your tailbone lengthening in the opposite direction. Your pubic bone should remain heavy, and your abdominals should be scooped inward.

4 Breathe out and gently lower your body back down to the ground. Maintain your strong centre and keep the muscles around your shoulder blades engaged, so that your shoulders don't hunch as you lower your upper body. Practise the whole exercise eight times.

1 Sit comfortably astride a small chair, facing its back, with your feet flat on the floor. Hold onto the back of the chair for support and make sure that both your "sit" bones are firmly planted on the seat of the chair. Pull up through your spine from your strong abdominals.

2 (*right*) Breathe in, then as you breathe out lift your left hand over your head, with the palm facing up. Avoid hunching your left shoulder. Breathe in again and breathe out to reach your arm further over to the right, bending your upper body sideways in line with your arm. Keep your bottom and hips still, firmly planted on the chair.

3 Breathe in and move your body upward a little, then breathe out to bring your left arm over your head, and reach to the right side again. Keep your abdominals engaged to prevent your lower back from arching. This time you are aiming to reach a little further over to the right.

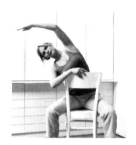

4 Breathe in to release the stretch and breathe out to repeat it one more time. Keep your head and neck in line with your spine, and avoid bending your neck toward the floor. Be sure to bend your body sideways and not forward – imagine you are moving between two sliding doors. Practise this exercise five times on each side.

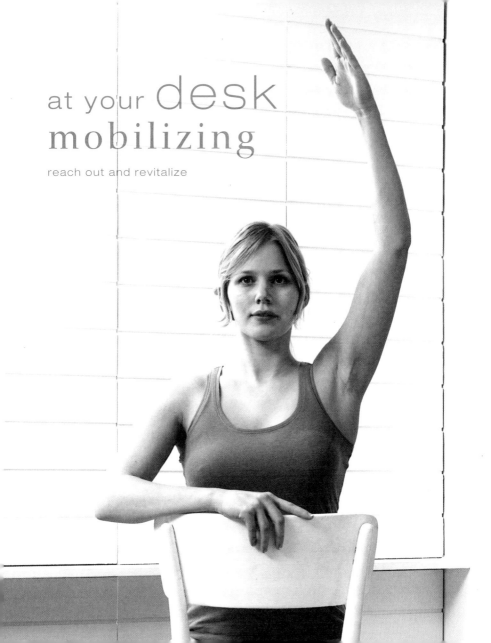

at your desk
mobilizing

reach out and revitalize

1 Sitting on your plane seat with your back as straight as possible, clasp both hands under your right thigh to support it. Lift your right foot away from the floor and straighten your leg slightly. Don't hunch your shoulders; all the movement should come from your leg.

2 (*right*) Point your foot softly away from your body, keeping your foot aligned with your knee and hip. Be careful not to twist your ankle so that your foot looks "sickled" or banana-shaped. "Flex" by bending your ankle so that the toes and ball of your foot pull toward your body and the heel reaches away. Repeat this nine times with your right foot, then change to your left leg and repeat ten times.

3 Pick up your right leg again. Point your toes away from your body, then pull them left so that your foot is slightly "sickled". Flex your ankle to bring your toes toward you and finally twist your foot outward. This completes a full clockwise circle.

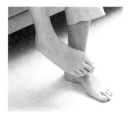

4 Repeat the clockwise circles nine times, then point your toes and turn your foot outward, pull your toes inward to flex your foot and sickle it to the left, to circle your foot anticlockwise ten times. Finally, complete ten clockwise and ten anticlockwise circles with your left foot.

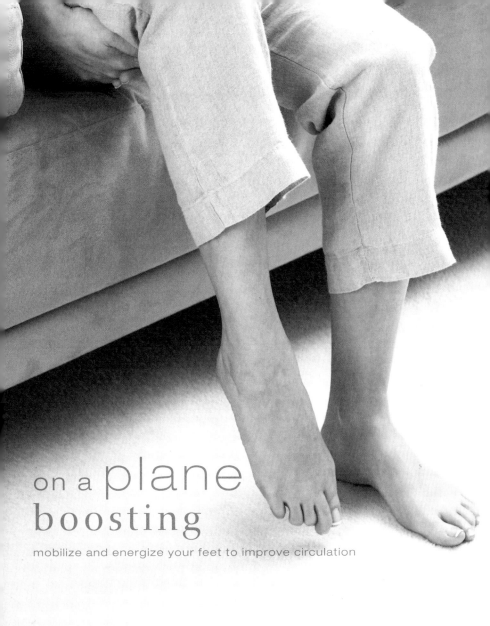

on a plane
boosting

mobilize and energize your feet to improve circulation

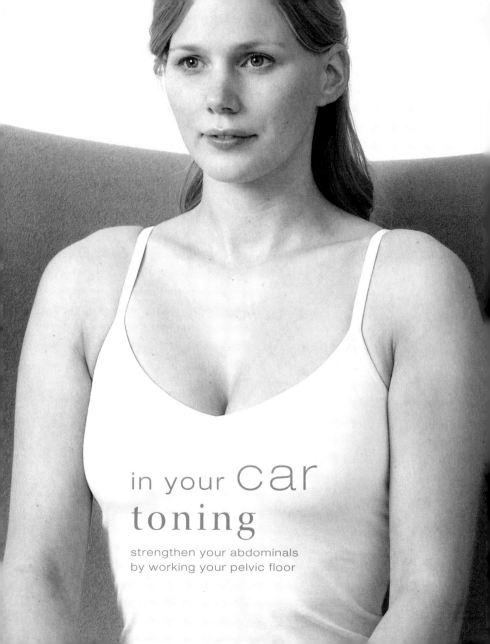

in your car
toning

strengthen your abdominals
by working your pelvic floor

1 Practise this exercise when your car is stationary, for example when you're stuck in traffic. Sit as upright as you can in your car seat, sitting high on your "sit" bones to ensure that your weight is evenly distributed on both buttocks. Relax your neck and shoulders. Breathe in.

2 Breathe out and slowly lift the muscles between your pubic bone and your tailbone. Imagine that you are trying to stop yourself urinating; this will help you to engage your pelvic floor muscles. If you can, hold these muscles for a count of five.

3 Breathe in and relax for a few seconds. As you breathe out, engage your pelvic floor muscles again. Imagine a zip fastening between your pubic bone and tailbone. In addition to this, draw your navel toward your lower spine so that you are hollowing your abdominal muscles.

4 Breathe in and relax again, then repeat the whole exercise a further two times. Working your pelvic floor muscles at the same time as your abdominals actually helps your abdominals to work more efficiently and become stronger.

1 Sit up on your "sit" bones with your legs stretched out in front of you. (You may find this easier if you sit on a rolled-up towel, or even a telephone directory, to help your lower spine to lengthen.) Your legs should be about 15cm (6in) apart, with your feet and toes relaxed.

2 (*right*) Breathe in to lift your arms out to the sides, palms facing out in line with your inner elbows. Pull your shoulder blades down into your back. Breathe out and twist your spine to the left so that you are facing your left leg. Your right arm will have moved toward your left leg and your left arm will be behind the line of your left shoulder.

3 Breathe in. As you breathe out reach toward your left foot. If you can, bring the outside of your right little finger to your left little toe. Lift and stretch your left arm behind you, without hunching your shoulder. Turn to look at your left hand.

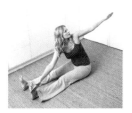

4 Breathe in as you hold this position, keeping your buttocks glued to the floor, and then breathe out to increase the stretch, reaching further past your left foot. Imagine resting your chest on your left thigh. Ensure your neck remains long. Breathe out and slowly return to sitting upright, then repeat the stretch on the other side, reaching forward with your left hand. Practise this exercise four times on each side.

in a hotel room
comforting
centre yourself to restore your sense of place

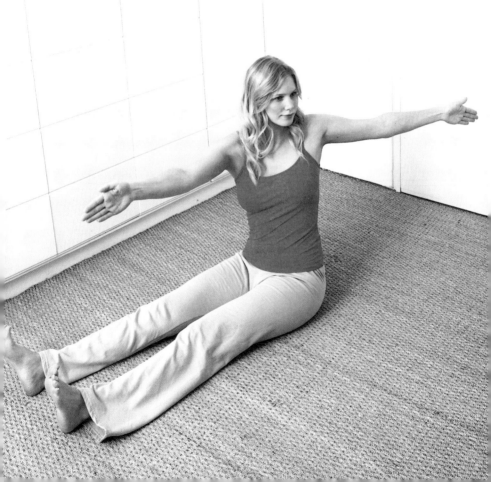

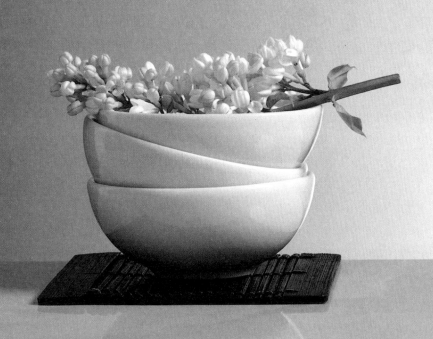

stress busters

You've probably noticed that your back, neck and shoulders tighten up when you're feeling under pressure. Stretch away your stress! Find some time to relax, practise some gentle Pilates exercises, and you'll soon discover that your mental and physical tensions melt away.

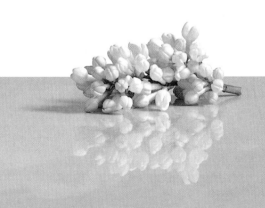

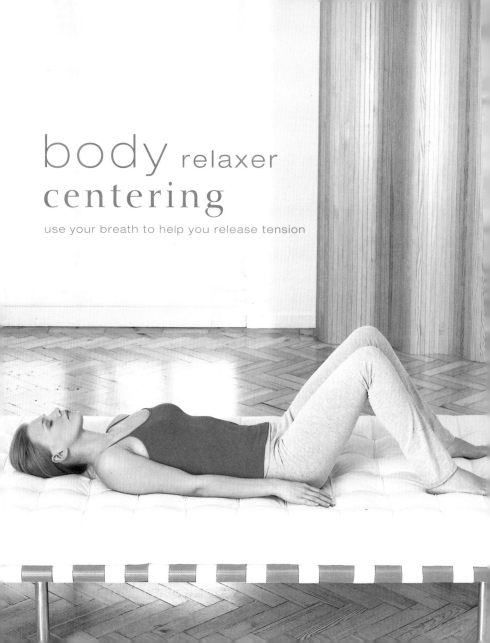

body relaxer
centering
use your breath to help you release tension

1 Lie on your back with your knees bent so that they are hip-width apart, or a little wider, if that's more comfortable. Keep your feet parallel. Be aware of the equal distribution of weight between the centre of your heels and the big and little toes of each foot.

2 If your neck feels strained, place a small pillow or paperback book under your head. Place your hands on your abdomen or by your sides and close your eyes. Take your focus to each part of your body in turn. Start with your head and face and work down your neck, shoulders, arms, torso, hips and legs to your feet.

3 Feel the weight of your head and allow tension to melt away from your forehead. Let your tongue relax down to the bottom of your mouth and release tension from your jaw. Feel the backs of your ribs and your spine melt into the surface beneath you. Release your thighs and soften the area around your hips.

4 Keep your breathing relaxed and flowing. Focus on releasing unwanted tension from your whole body, allowing your torso to widen, your spine to lengthen and your feet to feel grounded. As well as using this exercise to unwind, you can use it to start or finish any of the other exercises in the book.

67

neck reliever
unwinding

let your mind empty to free your neck

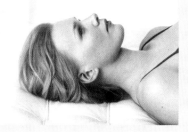 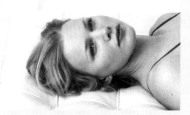

1 Lie on your back with your legs outstretched and completely relaxed, and your arms by your sides. Place a small cushion under your head if your neck feels strained. Release your neck and your jaw as much as possible. Relax your chest and allow your shoulder blades to melt downward. Breathe in.

2 As you breathe out, roll your head slowly to the right, allowing the weight of your head to govern the movement. Breathe in, bring your head back to the centre and pause for a moment. As you breathe out, roll your head to the left. Roll your head gently from side to side like this ten times.

68

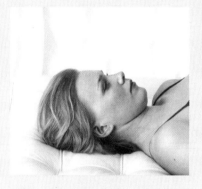

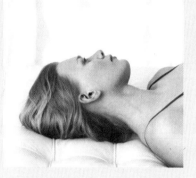

3 Breathe in and bring your head back to the centre. As you breathe out, slowly bring your chin toward your chest. Keep your head heavy and feel the back of your neck lengthening. Turn your head to your right and lift your chin so that you begin to circle your head clockwise.

4 Move your head in a small circle, being careful not to tip it too far back. Repeat nine times, making your circles small to begin with, then gradually increasing their size. Breathe in between circles. Keep your head heavy in order to release all the tension in your neck. Finish with ten anticlockwise circles.

69

1 (*right*) Lie on your back with your knees bent, feet placed hip-width apart and parallel. Raise your arms so that they are directly over your shoulders, with your palms facing each other and fingers relaxed. Feel your upper back widening and the tension in your shoulders releasing down into the floor. Relax your head and look toward the ceiling.

2 Breathe in and reach up with your left arm, lifting your shoulder off the floor. Lengthen your fingertips up as high as you can, so that your whole shoulder blade lifts off the floor, and you can feel a stretch in your upper back.

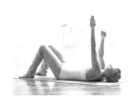

3 Breathe out and drop your shoulder back down to the floor. Feel the weight of your arm sinking into your shoulder joint. Breathe in and reach up with your right arm. Stretch as far up as you can, then breathe out to drop your shoulder blade back down to the floor.

4 Bring your attention to your abdominals, and pull them in to maintain stability in your pelvis. This will ensure that during the repetitions your spine is relaxed and doesn't twist. Your head will naturally move a little as you reach upward, but if you feel any discomfort, support your head with a small cushion. Practise this exercise five times with each arm.

shoulder loosener
reviving

unlock stress held in your shoulders

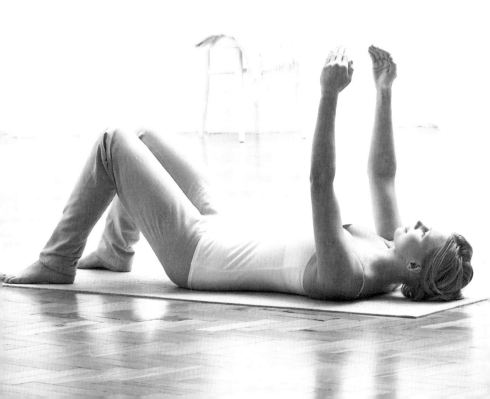

arm releaser
freeing

work with the full weight of gravity to help you relax

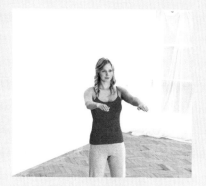 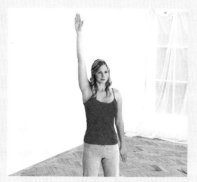

1 Stand with your feet placed hip-width apart and parallel. Visualize your head balancing lightly at the top of your spine. Relax your shoulders and drop your tailbone toward the floor. Gently pull in your abdominals, without altering the position of your pelvis. Breathe in and raise your arms to shoulder height, palms facing down.

2 Breathe out and lift your right arm up toward the ceiling, palm facing forward. At the same time lower your left arm down, palm facing back. Extend your fingers as far as you can, making sure both shoulders remain stable. Feel your arms growing longer, being careful not to tense your wrists.

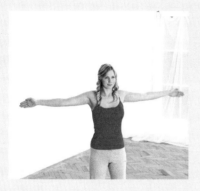 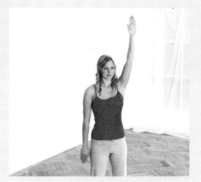

3 Breathe in as you move your right arm sideways and down, and lift your left arm sideways and up to shoulder height. Turn your left palm to face forward. Your shoulders should remain relaxed. Feel a long, relaxing stretch from one hand right across your chest to the other hand.

4 Breathe out and again move both hands in an arc shape, your right arm down toward the floor, palm facing back, and your left arm up, palm facing forward. Breathe in to bring both arms back to the starting position. Repeat five times on each side.

1 Kneel on all fours, with your hands directly under your shoulders, your knees directly under your hips and your head in line with your spine. Look down toward the floor. Relax your feet: you can support them with a small cushion if you prefer.

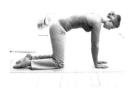

2 (*right*) Breathe in, and as you breathe out draw your abdominals upward and inward toward your spine. Arch your mid-back, and curl your tailbone under your hips. Relax your head down toward the floor, without over-stretching your neck. Pull your shoulder blades down toward your hips to prevent your shoulders from hunching.

3 Breathe in as you hold this position, being careful not to raise your shoulders or relax your stomach. As you breathe out, extend your tailbone then gradually lengthen your lower back, middle back, upper back, neck and head until you have returned to the starting position.

4 Breathe in and repeat the exercise, pressing down into your hands to help maintain stability in your shoulders. Ensure that your thighs don't move at all and your hips stay aligned over your knees. If your wrists feel strained, place a small cushion or slim paperback book under the heel of each hand. Practise this exercise eight times.

back soother
balancing

unwind with this liberating stretch

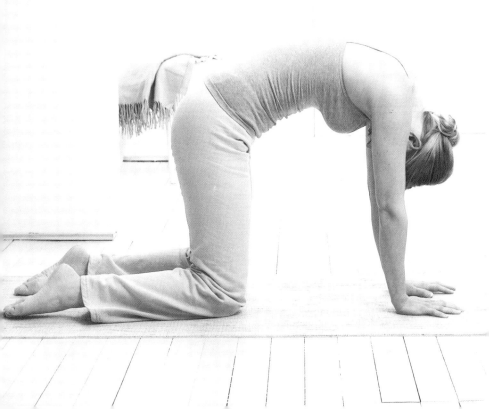

1 Lie on your back with your feet and knees placed wider than hip-width apart. Relax your arms out to the sides, just below shoulder height. Feel your whole spine lengthen and sense the floor supporting you. Relax your shoulders. Breathe in.

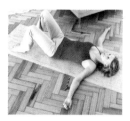

2 (*right*) As you breathe out, engage your abdominals and slowly roll your knees and hips to the right, turning your head to the left. At the same time, bring your right arm across your chest, so that it is slightly lower than your left arm. Drop your left knee toward your right heel until you feel a stretch through your left thigh and the front of your left hip.

3 Breathe in. Check that you have not arched your back or allowed your ribs to flare outward. Breathe out and pull in your abdominals to lift your legs and manoeuvre your body and right arm back to the starting position. Imagine each part of your body aligning in sequence: first your ribcage, then your waist, then your lower back and finally your legs.

4 Practise the whole exercise three more times rolling to the right, then four times rolling to the left. Take your knees and hips only a little way over to start with, and aim to roll further with each repetition. Eventually you are aiming to take both knees down to the floor.

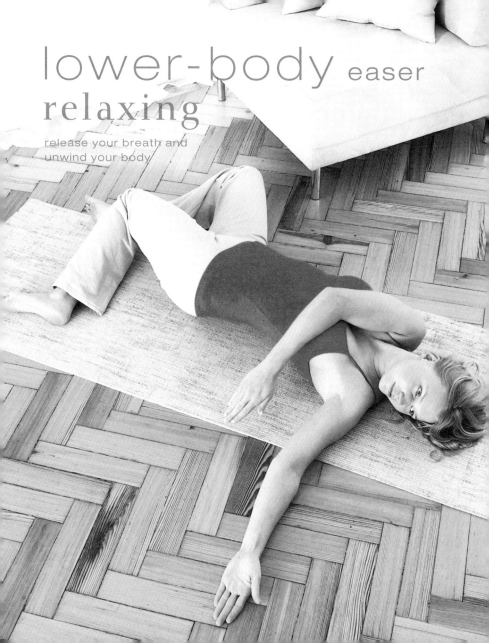

lower-body easer

relaxing

release your breath and
unwind your body

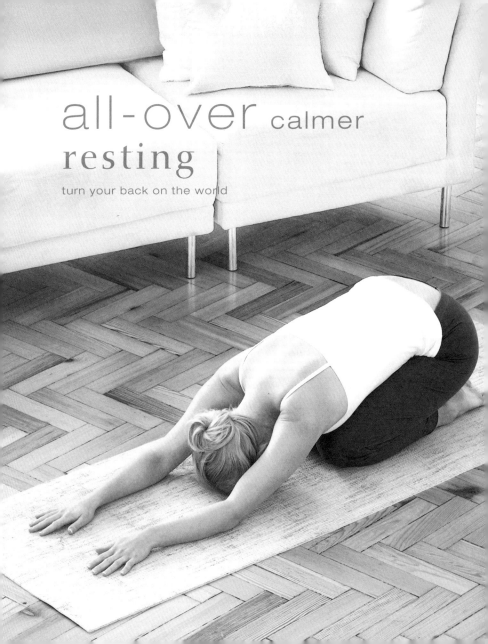

all-over calmer

resting

turn your back on the world

1 Sit back on your heels with your knees apart and your hands resting on your thighs. Breathe in. As you breathe out, bend forward from your hips. Stretch your arms forward as far as you can reach. Keep your buttocks and feet together; if it's more comfortable, you can place a small cushion between them.

2 Now bring your forearms to the floor and relax your neck. Keep your arms extended to give your body the maximum stretch. Close your eyes, breathe, rest and relax in this position for at least five breaths.

3 (*opposite*) If you can, bring your forehead to the floor between your arms, being careful not to lift your tailbone away from your heels. Place a small cushion under your head if that's more comfortable. Breathe deeply, imagining that your breath is expanding the back of your ribcage. Stay here for five breaths.

4 Bring your elbows back toward your knees. Breathe out, pulling in your abdominals, and slowly sit up. Visualize dropping your tailbone down and bringing your pubic bone forward. Rebuild your spine, vertebra by vertebra, until you are kneeling upright, and open your eyes.

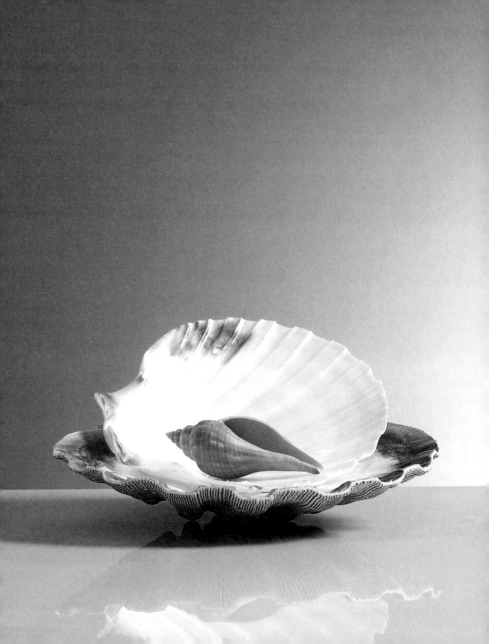

energy
boosters

Too worn out to go to the gym or for that power walk? Simply pick

two or three exercises from the following chapter to quickly and easily

revitalize your energy levels. You'll soon feel recharged – and you'll be

able to continue your day with a new lease of life!

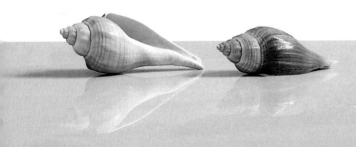

all-over energizer
restoring

focus your mind and body to lift your energy levels

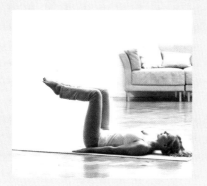 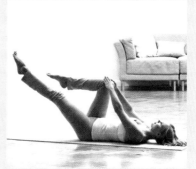

1 Lie on your back with both knees bent. Relax your arms down by your sides. Breathe in, and as you breathe out fold your right knee toward your chest, using your abdominals to keep your pelvis still. Imagine your thigh bone dropping into your hip. Lift your left knee. Place your feet together and allow your knees to open slightly.

2 Breathe in and place both hands on your right knee. As you breathe out, stretch your left leg diagonally away from you, and gently point your toes. Keep your abdominals strong to prevent your back from arching, and relax your neck and shoulders.

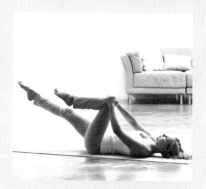

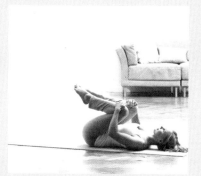

3 Breathe in as you bend your left leg toward your chest and breathe out to extend your right leg. Simultaneously, change the position of your hands so that they are holding your left knee. Keep your elbows open and your chest muscles soft.

4 Repeat steps 2 and 3 until you have practised the exercise six times with each leg. To finish, pull your knees into your chest to release your hips and lower back. Release your hands, and slowly replace your right and then your left foot on the floor.

83

tummy lifter
rejuvenating

increase your strength and stamina

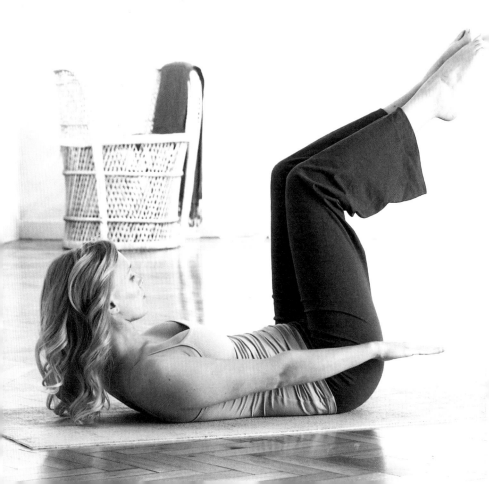

1 Lie on your back with both knees bent, feet placed hip-width apart. Rest your head on a small cushion if you need to, and extend your arms alongside your body, palms down. Keeping your feet and knees together, carefully bend your right and then your left knee in toward your chest. Lift your feet slightly higher than your knees.

2 Use your abdominals to connect your lower spine to the floor. Slide your shoulders down, and lift your arms so that they are level with your hips. If your lower back is uncomfortable, bring your knees a little closer to your chest, without lifting your tailbone. Lift your head, tucking in your chin to avoid straining your neck.

3 (*left*) Breathe in for five counts. As you breathe, move your arms up and down in a pumping action, co-ordinating the movements with your counts. As you inhale, imagine widening the back of your rib-cage. Breathe out for five counts, pumping your arms as before and focusing on scooping in your abdominals.

4 Begin by practising four sets of ten breaths, in for five counts and out for five. As you grow stronger, gradually build up to ten sets of ten breaths. While you move your arms, make sure they remain isolated from your shoulders. If your lower back begins to arch or ache, rest your legs on a chair or exercise ball.

85

1 Lie on the floor with your knees and feet together. Stretch your arms out to the sides at shoulder height, with your palms up. Relax your shoulders down into your back and allow your spine and arms to feel heavy and relaxed. Breathe in.

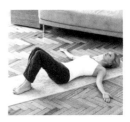

2 (*right*) Breathe out as you slowly roll your knees and hips a short distance over to the right, gently turning your head to the left. Use your abdominal muscles to peel your left hip, left buttock and the back of your left ribs away from the floor. Keep the outer edge of your right foot on the floor and allow your left foot to lift off, keeping your knees together. Stop if you feel your left shoulder begin to lift. Breathe in.

3 Breathe out and use your abdominals to return your knees, hips and feet to the starting position. Simultaneously turn your head to the centre. Keep your feet and knees together throughout steps 2 and 3: imagine that they form a single "leg".

4 Breathe in, and breathe out to roll to the left, turning your head to the right. Keep your abdominals pulled in throughout the exercise as you move your legs to ensure that your back does not arch. Practise the whole exercise five times on each side.

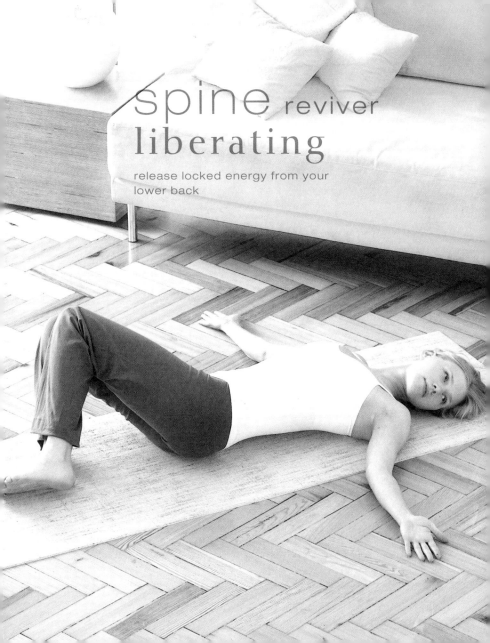

spine reviver
liberating

release locked energy from your
lower back

tummy refresher
stimulating

enliven your core and renew your body's energy

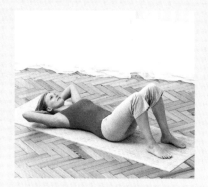

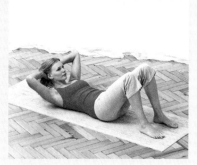

1 Lie on your back with both knees bent, feet placed hip-width apart. Interlace your fingers and bring your hands to support the back of your head. Slide your shoulders down into your back and allow your elbows to lift slightly so that you can see them in your peripheral vision. Breathe in.

2 Breathe out and, engaging your abdominals, slowly curl your head and shoulders away from the floor. Tuck in your chin a little, as if you were holding a small ball beneath it. Soften your chest muscles and keep your pelvis still. Look down between your knees.

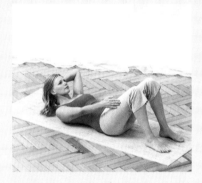

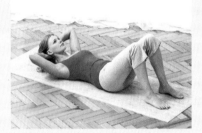

3 Keeping your tailbone heavy and your abdominals strong, breathe in and release your right hand from your head, reaching it forward toward your right knee. Be careful not to tense the fronts of your hips – imagine trying to keep a marble balanced on your navel. Initiate the "pull" from your abdominals and pelvic floor muscles.

4 Breathe out, replace your right hand and slowly lower your body to the ground. Repeat the curl-up, this time reaching forward with your left hand. Repeat the curl-ups eight times. Practise each curl-up slowly with control, leading with alternate arms. Finally, allow your head to sink into your hands.

1 Lie on your back with your knees bent and your knees and feet together. Clasp your hands lightly behind your head and lift your elbows so that they are within your peripheral vision. Breathe in, and as you breathe out lift your right leg toward

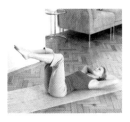

your chest, followed by your left leg. Your thighs form a right angle to your body and your feet are together, slightly higher than your knees.

2 (*right*) Breathe in again, and breathe out to slowly curl your head up from the floor. Keep your chin gently tucked in to isolate your head from your shoulders, and keep the back of your neck long. As you curl up, straighten your legs as much as you can, softly pointing your toes.

3 Check that your abdominals remain strong, helping to keep the whole length of your spine anchored to the floor. Breathe in, still engaging your abdominals, and lower your head back down to the floor. Simultaneously bend your knees toward your chest.

4 Repeat steps 2, 3 and 4, taking your legs slightly further away from your body this time. As you get stronger you will be able to take your legs further and further down. Repeat the whole exercise. Start with five repetitions then, when you are used to it, increase to ten repetitions.

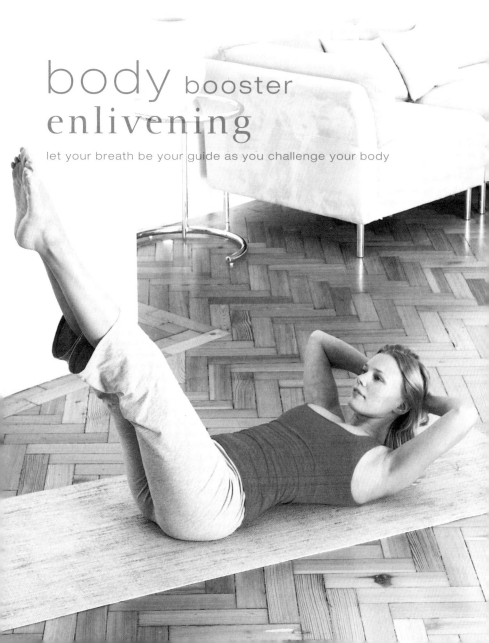

body booster
enlivening

let your breath be your guide as you challenge your body

thigh invigorator
stabilizing

revive your legs by working with gravity

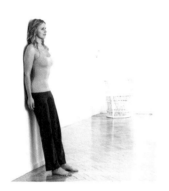

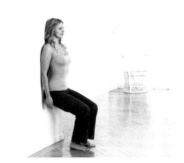

1 Stand with your back against a wall and your feet hip-width apart and about 15cm (6in) or your own foot's length away from the wall. Support yourself by leaning into the wall, but don't force your head back.

2 Breathe in and lengthen up through your spine as much as possible. As you breathe out, slowly bend your knees until your thighs are almost parallel with the floor. Keep your knees in line with your middle toes and your heels placed firmly on the ground.

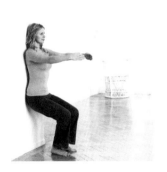

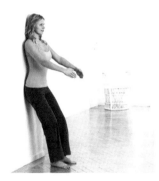

3 Pull in your abdominals and breathe in as you lift your arms to just below shoulder height, palms facing each other. Relax your shoulders. Visualize your tailbone lengthening toward the floor and your head moving up toward the ceiling, as if your spine is being pulled in both directions.

4 Breathe out and start to straighten your knees. Slowly slide up the wall again, keeping your back straight and abdominals pulled in. At the same time, slowly lower your arms. Practise this exercise eight times.

1 Lie on your left side with both knees bent. Your spine should be in a straight line; you can lie against a wall to check your alignment. Extend your left arm under your ear and place a folded towel between your ear and your shoulder. Place your right hand lightly on the floor in front of your chest for support. Your right shoulder should be directly over your left shoulder and your right hip should be over your left hip.

2 Draw in your abdominals and lift the left side of your waist to prevent it sinking into the floor. Breathe in and extend your right leg away from you, lifting it to level with your hip. Flex your ankle.

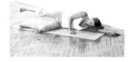

3 (*right*) Breathe out and lift your leg to about 15cm (6in) above hip height, keeping it straight so that the outer thigh muscle works. Be careful not to take your leg behind you. Keep your abdominals strong to stabilize your pelvis and prevent your back from arching.

4 Breathe in to lower your leg back to hip height. Raise and lower your leg eight times, co-ordinating the movements with your breathing. As you lift, imagine your leg lengthening out from your heel. Finally, bend your right leg to rest on top of your left leg. Turn onto your right side, and repeat the whole exercise with your left leg.

outer-thigh lifter
boosting
strengthen and recharge your legs

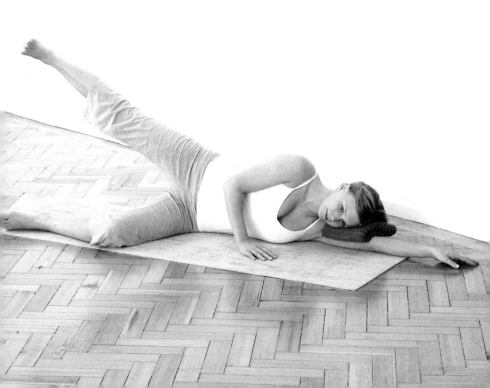

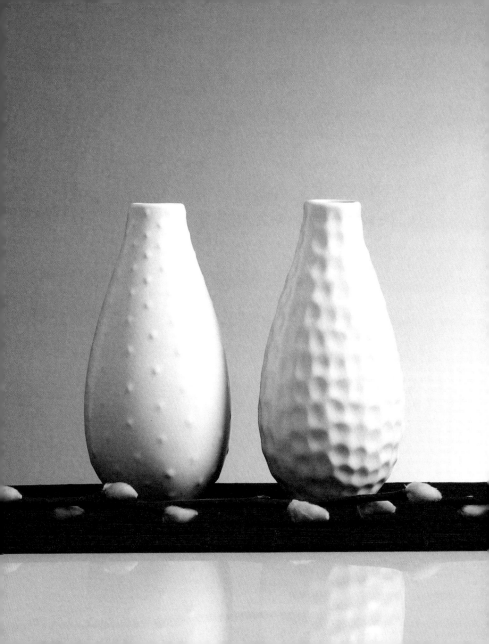

toners and strengtheners

To achieve lean muscles, you need the perfect balance of tone and

strength. But you don't have to do endless hours of weight training in

the gym: in this chapter there's an exercise to tone every part of your

body, all within the comfort of your own home!

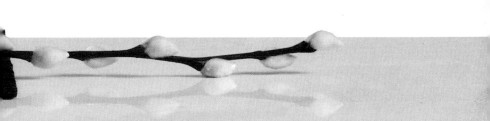

body toner
anchoring

strengthen your centre to bring yourself back into balance

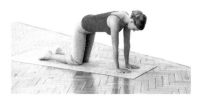

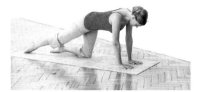

1 Kneel on all fours, with your hands directly beneath your shoulders and your knees directly beneath your hips. Make sure your head and spine are aligned. Breathe in and imagine your spine lengthening from the top of your head to the tip of your tailbone.

2 Breathe out, engaging your abdominals. Slide your right foot along the floor and straighten your leg in line with your hip. Your back and pelvis should remain still and your eyes should look toward the floor. Keep your shoulders relaxed down into your back.

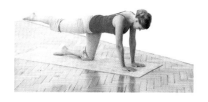

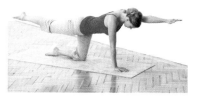

3 Breathe in. Maintaining a stable pelvis, carefully lift your right leg to hip height. Softly point your toes. Your leg should feel long. Keep your abdominals strong to help you to maintain your balance and to prevent your lower back from dipping.

4 Breathe out and lift your left arm to shoulder height, without hunching your shoulder. Feel your arm lengthen, but don't over-reach. Lift your abdominals to help relieve the weight on your left knee and right hand. Breathe in to lower your right leg and left arm simultaneously. Practise this exercise four times on each side.

1 Lie on your stomach. Extend your arms above your head, a little wider than shoulder-width apart. Stretch your legs out a little wider than hip-width apart. If your nose feels squashed, rest your forehead on a small cushion. Breathe in.

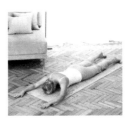

2 (*right*) Breathe out as you lift your left arm and right leg no more than 10cm (4in) off the floor. Imagine you have a marble under your navel, and you are trying to draw your navel away from it; your aim is to engage your abdominals to stabilize your shoulders and pelvis.

3 Hold this position and breathe in. Imagine sending your breath to the back of your rib-cage rather than lifting the top of your shoulders. Visualize your spine lengthening away from your strong centre. Keep both your hips and your pubic bone heavy on the floor.

4 Breathe out as you lower your arm and leg slowly with control, still maintaining the stretch. Repeat the exercise with your right arm and left leg. If you want to work your upper back muscles a little more, try lifting your head about 5cm (2in), keeping your eyes down on the floor. Practise this exercise four times on each side.

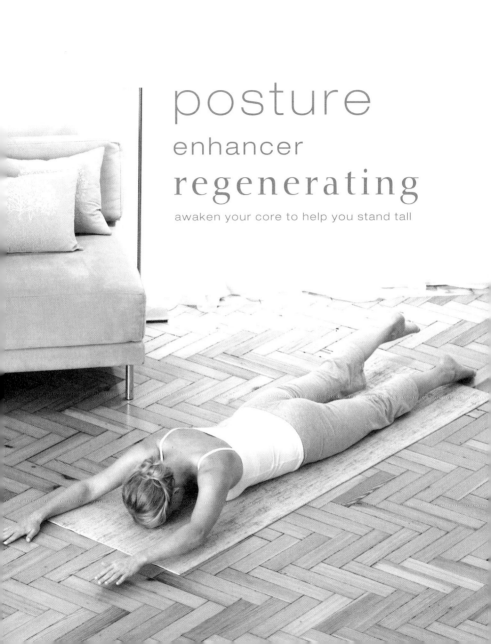

posture
enhancer
regenerating
awaken your core to help you stand tall

waist tightener
toning
twist and stretch to rediscover your hourglass shape

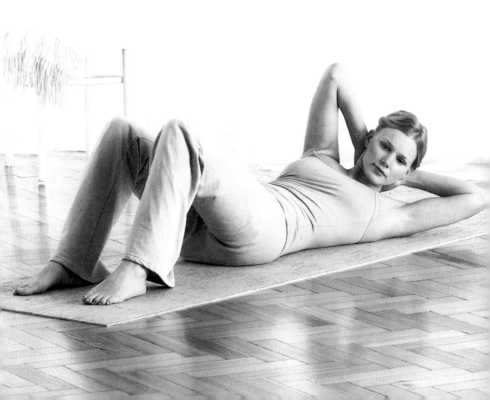

1 Lie on your back with your knees bent, feet placed hip-width apart. Interlace your fingers and support the back of your head with your hands. Lift your elbows away from the floor so that they are within your peripheral vision. Breathe in.

2 Breathe out, engage your abdominals and pelvic floor muscles and curl up. Rotate your torso so that you are taking your right shoulder toward the outside of your left knee. Keep your right hip grounded and release the fronts of both hips.

3 (*left*) Breathe in to hold this position for a moment, feeling your right ribs pulling diagonally toward your left hip. Ensure that your hands are not pulling your head forward – they should just be cradling it. Keep your right elbow open, moving forward solely from your shoulder.

4 Breathe out and lower your body and head back to the floor. Relax both shoulders, but keep your elbows level with the fronts of your ears, ready for your next curl-up on the right side. Repeat the whole exercise five times on each side.

1 (*right*) Sit on the floor with your knees bent and feet hip-width apart. Pull up through your abdominals to help you straighten your back and sit high on your "sit" bones. Lift your arms in front of you to just below shoulder height, with your palms facing each other. Breathe in.

2 Breathe out and start to tilt your pelvis forward so that your pubic bone comes up toward the ceiling. Be careful not to drop your chin or round your shoulders. Keep your shoulders relaxed to prevent your upper back from hunching.

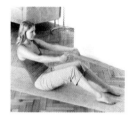

3 Still breathing out, continue to curl your lower spine and hollow your abdominals until you are sitting back on your tailbone. Curl backward a little further. Release the muscles around your hips, and be careful not to poke your head forward from your neck. Breathe in.

4 Breathe out and begin to move your body forward, back on to your "sit" bones. Scoop your abdominals inward, so that you come up with your back slightly rounded. Keep your arms straight, but avoid pulling your body forward with them. Practise this exercise eight times.

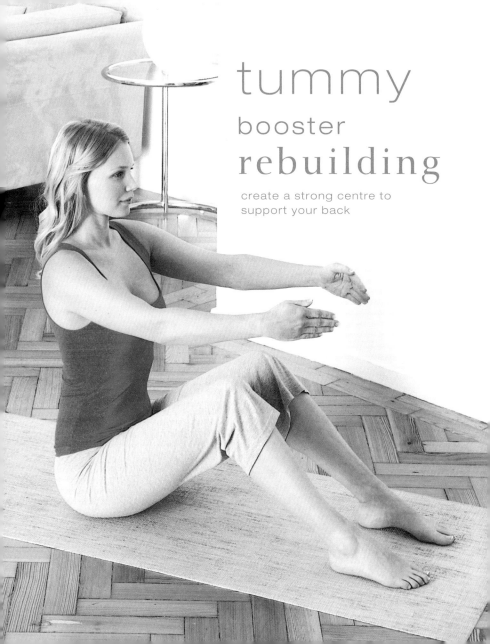

tummy
booster
rebuilding

create a strong centre to
support your back

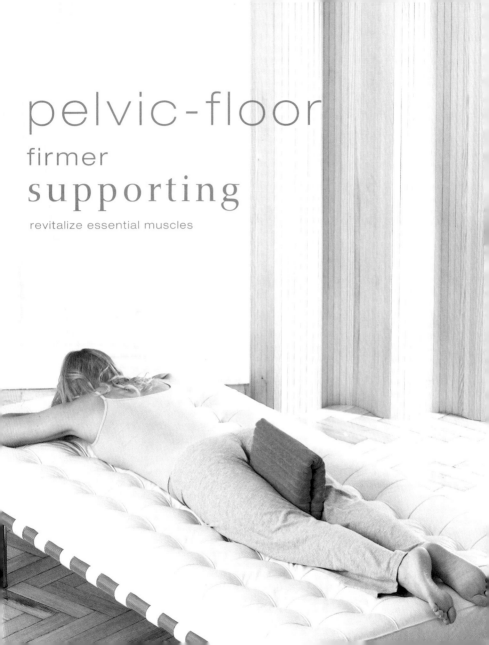

pelvic-floor

firmer

supporting

revitalize essential muscles

1 Lie on your front with your legs relaxed, your toes together and your heels apart. Place a folded towel between the tops of your thighs. Place your right hand on top of your left and rest your forehead on your folded hands. Relax your neck and shoulders. Breathe in deeply and lengthen through your spine.

2 (*opposite*) Breathe out, and engage your pelvic floor and abdominal muscles. Bring your heels together and push your big toes apart, turning your legs out from your hips. This movement will draw your inner thighs together so that you are gently squeezing the folded towel. Hold this position for a count of five.

3 Visualize a magnet under each hip bone and your pubic bone, keeping them anchored to the surface beneath you. Be particularly careful that your feet don't lift, as this may strain your lower back. As you squeeze the towel, relax any tension in your shoulders, neck and jaw.

4 Breathe in and release first your inner thighs, then your buttocks, followed by your lower abdominals and finally your pelvic floor muscles. Rest for a few breaths, then repeat the whole exercise four times.

107

tummy flattener
firming

build a washboard stomach

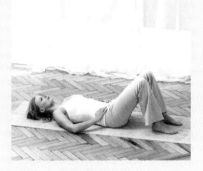

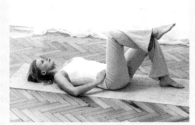

1 Lie on your back with your knees bent and your feet placed hip-width apart. Place your hands on the fronts of your hips to ensure that your pelvis stays in a stable position throughout this exercise. Relax your shoulders and neck. Breathe in.

2 Breathe out, engaging your abdominals, and lift your right leg, keeping your knee bent. Bring your leg to a right angle with your body. Your knee should be directly over your hip and your foot in line with your knee. Softly point your toes. Imagine your thigh bone dropping down into your hip and anchoring there. Breathe in.

108

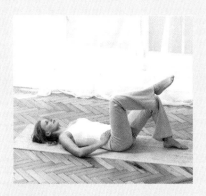

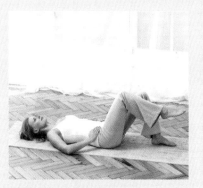

3 Breathe out and turn your leg out so that your right knee moves out to the side and your right foot moves toward your left knee. Make sure this movement is initiated from your hip joint, not from your knee.

4 Breathe in and return your leg to the central position in step 2. Use your hands to check the stability of your pelvis again. Breathe out and lower your leg carefully back to the floor, using your lower abdominals to prevent your back from arching. Practise this exercise eight times with each leg.

109

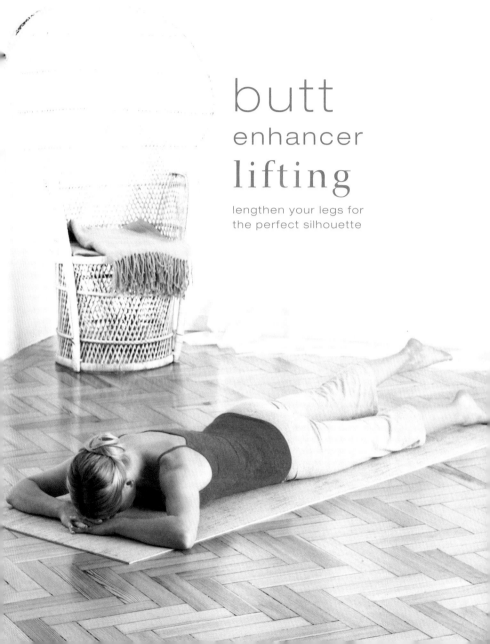

butt
enhancer
lifting

lengthen your legs for
the perfect silhouette

1 Lie on your front with your hands folded in front of you. Rest your head on your hands. Place your legs shoulder-width apart, and slightly turn them out from your hips by bringing your heels toward each other. Relax your shoulders and your upper back. Engage your abdominals to stabilize your pelvis. Breathe in.

2 (*opposite*) Breathe out as you lift your right leg no more than 5cm (2in) away from the floor, being careful not to lift your right hip or tense your shoulders. Stretch your leg, lengthening it away from the hip socket, and softly point your toes. Breathe in as you hold this position.

3 As you breathe out, slowly circle your leg five times clockwise and five times anticlockwise. Initiate each circle from the top of your thigh bone rather than from your foot. Keep your abdominals strong and feel your right buttock working. If you run out of breath while doing the circles, take another breath in.

4 Breathe out again and carefully lower your leg to the floor. Then repeat steps 2 and 3 with your left leg. The key to this exercise lies not in lifting your leg high, but in lengthening your leg away from a stable pelvis; small movements are more effective. Practise this exercise eight times with each leg.

1 Lie on your right side with both knees bent, your thighs at a 45-degree angle to your body and your feet directly below your buttocks. Extend your right arm under your ear and place a small cushion or folded towel between your shoulder 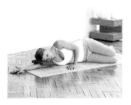 and your ear. Ensure that your left hip and shoulder are aligned directly over your right. Place your left hand in front of your chest. Breathe in.

2 (*right*) Breathe out and lift the right side of your waist away from the floor, enough that there would be space for you to slide your fingers underneath. Rotate your thigh from within your left hip and, keeping your pelvis still and your feet connected, lift your right knee away from your left. Engage your abdominals to help make this easier.

3 Breathe in as you hold this position and then breathe out and lift your left knee higher, if you can do so without moving your hip. This will increase the work on your outer hip and outer thigh. If you're having trouble, try placing your left hand on your hip to keep it still.

4 Breathe in and lower your knee with control, pressing into your left hand to ensure that your left hip doesn't pull forward and over-balance you. Repeat this movement seven more times, then roll over to your left side and practise the exercise eight times with your right leg.

hip toner
smoothing

refine your curves while you free your back

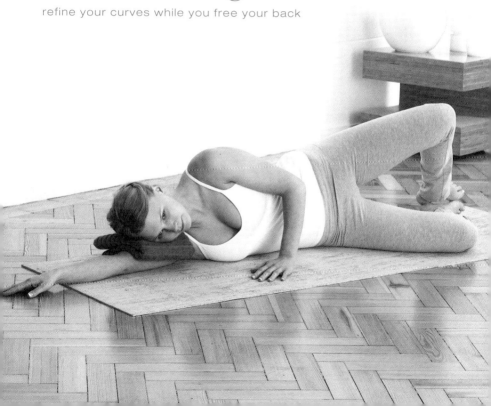

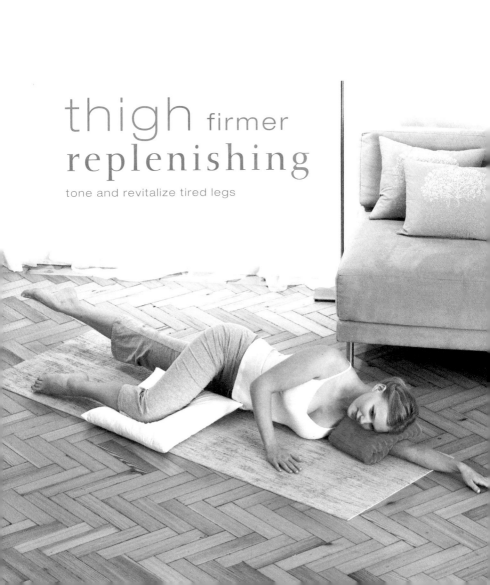

thigh firmer
replenishing

tone and revitalize tired legs

1 Lie on your left side. Bend your right knee to a 90-degree angle, and rest it on a cushion. Extend your left arm and place a folded towel between your left ear and shoulder. Place your right palm on the floor for support. Lengthen your spine and move your left leg slightly forward from your hip. Breathe in.

2 (*opposite*) Breathe out and lift your left leg, turning it out from your hip so that you feel the top of your inner thigh working. Stretch your leg and softly point your toes. Engage your abdominals to lift the left side of your waist. Ensure that you are turning your leg out from the hip and not twisting from your knee.

3 Breathe in and hold this position. Breathe out and lift your leg a little further, then pulse it up and down five times to challenge and tone the muscles of your inner thigh. Keep your pelvis still and your upper body open and relaxed.

4 Breathe in and lower your leg with control. Repeat steps 2 and 3 seven more times, then roll over to your right side and practise the whole exercise eight times with your right leg. For a different effect, experiment with flexing your foot instead of pointing it. You may feel your inner thigh working even harder.

hamstring helper
limbering

restore suppleness for greater strength

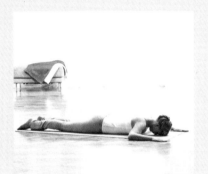 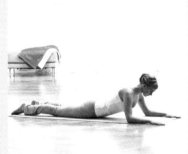

1 Lie on your front with your hands placed on the floor in line with your elbows, a little wider than shoulder-width apart. If your nose feels squashed, rest your forehead on a small cushion or, if it's more comfortable, turn your head to the side. Stretch your legs, and place them hip-width apart. Engage your abdominals and breathe in.

2 Breathe out and gently push down onto your forearms to raise your upper body off the floor. Slide your shoulders down into your back and keep your neck long. Look down between your hands. Keep your chest and abdominals lifted. If you find this position strains your back, rest your head down in the starting position.

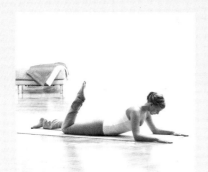

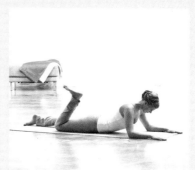

3 Gently point your toes. Breathe in, bend your knee and kick your right leg toward your buttocks. Make sure both your hips stay in contact with the floor; the movement should come from your knee. Breathe out and release your leg slightly toward the floor.

4 Breathe in, flex your ankle and repeat the kick. Breathe out and relax your foot, then extend your leg back down on the floor. Breathe in and repeat steps 3 and 4 with your left leg. Alternate legs until you have practised this exercise eight times with each leg.

117

1 Lie on your front with your forehead on the floor. If your nose feels squashed, place a folded towel or a small cushion under your head. Stretch your legs hip-width apart. Place your hands on either side of your shoulders, with your elbows

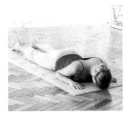

close to your body and fingers pointing forward. Make sure that your pubic bone and hip bones are in contact with the floor. Breathe in.

2 (*right*) Breathe out and, imagining that you are rolling a marble forward with your nose, gradually lift your forehead, nose, chin and then shoulders. Using your stomach and back muscles, lift your torso – your hands are just there for support. Look down to avoid over-extending your neck. Your arms are now half-stretched.

3 Breathe in and hold this position, gently turning your head from side to side to release any tension in your neck. Roll your shoulders back to open your chest. Engage your abdominals: imagine that you have a zip fastening from your pubic bone up to your breastbone.

4 Breathe out and bend your elbows to slowly lower your body to the floor. How high you lift in this exercise will depend on your spine's flexibility: start gradually and always engage your abdominals before you come up. Practise the whole exercise eight times.

118

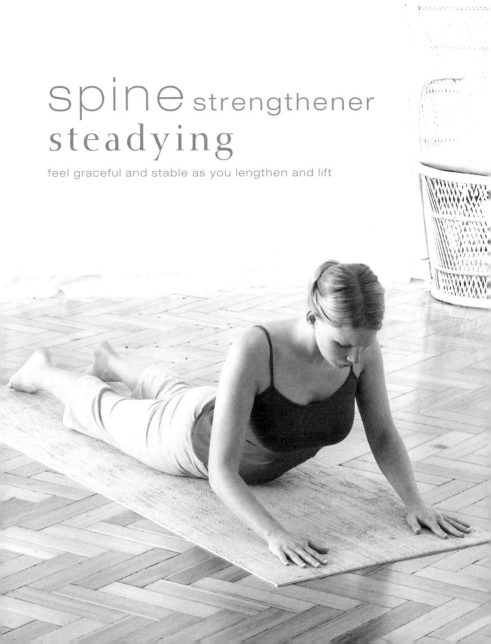

spine strengthener
steadying

feel graceful and stable as you lengthen and lift

back rebuilder
lengthening

stretch your back to improve your posture

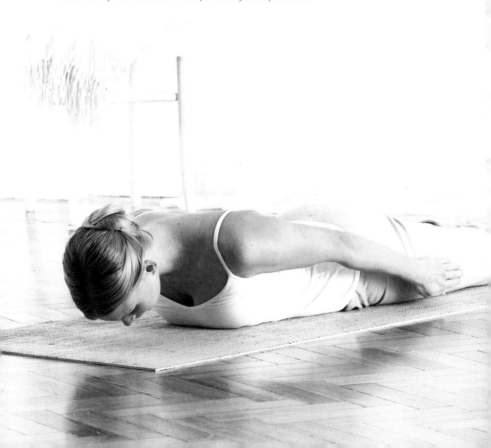

1 Lie on your front. If your nose feels squashed, rest your forehead on a small pillow or folded towel to help you breathe more easily. Lengthen your arms down at your sides, palms facing up. Place your legs together and relax your buttocks. Engage your abdominals. Breathe in.

2 Breathe out and tuck your chin under slightly as you lift your head away from the floor. Slide your shoulders down into your back. At the same time, turn your palms in to face your thighs, lifting your arms no more than 5cm (2in) off the floor, and lengthen your fingers down toward the sides of your knees.

3 (*left*) Breathe in as you hold this position, lifting your abdominals away from the floor while keeping your pubic bone and hip bones down. Slightly squeeze your inner thighs and buttocks and imagine lengthening your head away from your tailbone. Keep your eyes on the floor to avoid tipping your head back.

4 Breathe out and lower your head, relaxing your arms and shoulders. Allow your legs and buttocks to soften and relax, and release your neck, shoulders and arms, too. Rest for a few breaths, then breathe in to repeat. Practise the whole exercise eight times.

1 Lie on your front. If your nose feels squashed, rest your forehead on a small cushion or folded towel to help you breathe more easily. Your arms are down by your sides, palms facing up. Stretch your legs and place them hip-width apart. Relax your buttocks and check that your hip bones are level and in contact with the floor. Breathe in.

2 Breathe out and lift your arms about 10cm (4in) off the floor, stretching your fingers. Be careful not to lock your elbows, or "pinch" your shoulder blades together. Keep your abdominals strong to support your lower back. Breathe in.

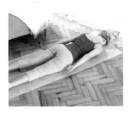

3 (*right*) Breathe out as you pulse your arms upward eight times. With each lift, imagine lengthening your arms and fingers away from your shoulders. Keep your shoulders stable and allow your head to relax completely so that your neck is not strained.

4 Breathe in and lower your arms, without letting your shoulders collapse forward. Repeat the movement eight times. Ensure that the only parts of your body that move are your arms. If you wish, you can use some light hand-weights to increase the efficacy of this exercise.

upper-arm
restorer
enhancing

rejuvenate lazy muscles and restore definition

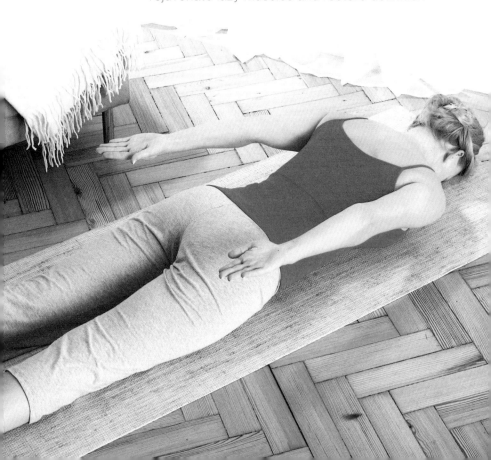

everyday sequences

If you are have a little more time for your Pilates practice, why not use these menus to select the best exercises for you – calming or energizing, toning or strengthening. You can practise these sequences in any suitable location.

half-hour unwinder	half-hour calmer	half-hour strenghener
66 body relaxer	42 in your bedroom	106 pelvic-floor firmer
68 neck reliever	48 in your bathroom	98 body toner
44 on your sofa	60 in your car	88 tummy refresher
36 before a meeting	76 lower-body easer	110 butt enhancer
24 lunchtime stretch	72 arm releaser	62 in a hotel room
30 bedtime wind-down	78 all-over calmer	92 thigh invigorator

one hour de-stress

26 afternoon uplifter
22 morning wake-up
48 in your bathroom
58 on a plane
30 bedtime wind-down
56 at your desk
44 on your sofa
74 back soother
42 in your bedroom
70 shoulder loosener
68 neck reliever
66 body relaxer

one hour tone-up

32 lazy weekend
34 before a night out
50 in the park
88 tummy refresher
94 outer-thigh lifter
38 at a conference
46 in your dining room
90 body booster
122 upper-arm restorer
110 butt enhancer
118 spine strengthener
112 hip toner

one hour energy booster

88 tummy refresher
86 spine reviver
82 all-over energizer
90 body booster
84 tummy lifter
104 tummy booster
100 posture enhancer
106 pelvic-floor firmer
92 thigh invigorator
102 waist tightener
94 outer-thigh lifter
114 thigh firmer

index

abdominal muscles
  core 8
  strengthening 11
  toning 60–1
  weakness in 11
activating 22–3
afternoon uplifter 26–7
alignment 13
all-over calmer 78–9
all-over energizer 82–3
anchoring 98–9
arms
  releaser 72–3
  upper-arm restorer 122–3

back
  core stability, effect of 8
  loosening 22–3
  pain 10–11
  rebuilder 120–1
  soother 74–5
  spine reviver 86–7
  spine strengthener 118–19
balancing 38–9, 74–5
bathroom, exercise in 48–9

beach, exercise on 54–5
bedroom, exercise in 42–3
bedtime wind–down 30–1
body booster 90–1
body relaxer 66–7
body toner 98–9
boosting 94–5
breathing
  correct 15–16
  exhalation 16
  inhalation 16
  lateral 15–16
  principle of Pilates, as 14
  thoracic 14–15
butt enhancer 110–11

car, exercise in 60–1
centering 14, 66–7
circulation, boosting 58–9
comforting 62–63
concentration 13
conference, exercise at 38–9
contraindications 16
co-ordination 14
core stability 8

desk, exercise at 56–7
dining room, exercise in 46–7

eight principles of Pilates
  alignment 13
  breathing 14
  centering 14
  concentration 13
  co-ordination 14
  flowing movements 14
  relaxation 13
  stamina 14–15
energizing 34–5
energy boosters
  all-over energizer 82–3
  body booster 90–1
  outer-thigh lifter 94–5
  spine reviver 86–7
  thigh invigorator 92–3
  tummy lifter 84–5
  tummy refresher 88–9
energy boosting 26–7, 81, 125
enhancing 122–3
enlivening 90–1
evening de-stress 28–9

everyday sequences 124–5
exhalation 16
exhilarating 50–4

firming 108–9
flexibility 10
flowing movements 14,
  32–3
focusing 36–7
freeing 72–3

half-hour exercises 124
hamstring helper 116–17
hip toner 112–13
hotel room, exercise in
  62–3

inhalation 16
invigorating 26–7

lazy weekend 32–3
leg stretch 28–9
lengthening 120–1
liberating 86–7
lifting 110–11

limbering 116–17
lower body easer 76–7
lunchtime stretch 24–5

meeting, exercise before
  36–7
mobility 10
mobilizing 56–7
morning wake–up 22–3

neck
  pain 10
  reliever 68–9
nurturing 54–5

one hour exercises 125
outer-thigh uplifter 94–5

park, exercise in 50–4
pelvic-floor firmer 106–7
Pilates
  benefits of 10
  contraindications 16
  efficacy of 7–8
  eight principles of 13–15

meaning 6–7
  versatility 19
Pilates, Joseph 6–7
plane, exercise on 58–9
posture 10
  enhancing 100–1
  muscles, endurance 14

rebuilding 104–5
refreshing 44–5, 114–15
regenerating 100–1
rejuvenating 84–5
relaxation 13
relaxing 42–3, 76–7
releasing 24–5
replenishing 114–15
resting 78–9
restoring 82–3
reviving 70–1

shoulder
  loosener 70–1
  pain 10
smoothing 112–13
sofa, exercise on 44–5

soothing 30–1

spine

  reviver 86–7

  strengthener 118–19

stabilizing 92–3

stamina 14–15

steadying 118–19

stimulating 88–9

strengthening 32–3, 118–19

  half-hour 124

stress

  one hour de-stress 125

  releasing 24–5

  stretching away 65

stress busters

  all-over calmer 78–9

arm releaser 72–3

back soother 74–5

body relaxer 66–7

lower-body easer 76–7

neck reliever 68–9

shoulder loosener 70–1

supporting 106–7

tensions, freeing 13, 30–1

thighs

  firmer 114–15

  invigorator 92–3

  outer-thigh uplifter 94–5

tone and strength 97

toning 60–1, 102–3

  one hour tone-up 125

tummy

  booster 104–5

  flattener 108–9

  lifter 84–5

  refresher 88–9

unwinding 28–9, 48–9, 68–9

  half-hour 124

uplifting 46–7

upper-arm restorer 122–3

users of Pilates 7–8

waist

  tightener 102–3

acknowledgments

author's acknowledgments

I would like to thank Ann Baggaley, Grace Cheetham, Jantje Doughty, Zoë Fargher, Kate Mahoney, Manisha Patel and Jules Selmes.

publisher's acknowledgments

Duncan Baird Publishers would like to thank model Kate Mahoney, hair and make-up artist Tinks Reding, and photographer's assistant Adam Giles.